Abdominal
X-rays
Made Easy

This book is dedicated to my mother, Lucy M. R. Begg

Front cover: Gross small bowel obstruction

For Churchill Livingstone:

Commissioning Editor: Laurence Hunter
Project Editor: Janice Urquhart
Project Controller: Frances Affleck
Design direction: Erik Bigland
Page layout: Jim Farley

Abdominal X-Rays Made Easy

James D. Begg MB BS FRCR

Consultant Radiologist,
Royal Victoria Hospital,
Dundee
and Honorary Senior Lecturer in
Diagnostic Radiology,
University of Dundee,
Scotland, UK

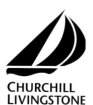

**CHURCHILL
LIVINGSTONE**

EDINBURGH LONDON NEW YORK PHILADELPHIA ST LOUIS SYDNEY TORONTO 1999

CHURCHILL LIVINGSTONE
An imprint of Elsevier Science Limited

First published 1999

ISBN 0 443 06205 6
  Reprinted 2001, 2002
International Student Edition ISBN 0 443 06206 4
  Reprinted 2000, 2001, 2002

British Library Cataloguing in Publication Data
A catalogue record for this book is available from the British
Library.

Library of Congress Cataloging in Publication Data
A catalog record for this book is available from the Library of
Congress.

Medical knowledge is constantly changing. As new information
becomes available, changes in treatment, procedures, equipment
and the use of drugs become necessary. The author and the
publishers have, as far as it is possible, taken care to ensure that the
information given in this text is accurate and up to date. However,
readers are strongly advised to confirm that the information,
especially with regard to drug usage, complies with current
legislation and standards of practice.

Printed in China by RDC Group Limited
C/03/04

Preface

The successful interpretation of all X-rays boils down to obeying a few simple rules and *knowing what you are looking for*. However, you must first overcome your feelings of a lack of knowledge and fear of making a mistake in trying to sort out the apparently overwhelming jumble of visual information which constitutes the abdominal X-ray.

Normal structures may masquerade as abnormalities and the way the film was taken, e.g. erect or supine, may grossly mislead the doctor into easy misinterpretation if this is not fully appreciated; which in turn can lead to the death of a patient, e.g. in a missed pneumoperitoneum.

For senior medical students such films loom large in the mind in the context of final examinations and future post-qualification responsibilities. This book therefore is designed to address both of these needs as well as being a useful reference for those about to face higher examinations in medicine and surgery. It should also be of value to colleagues interested in the subject in professions allied to medicine such as nursing and radiography.

Looking at X-rays is an *active* not a passive process. It is not sufficient to sit back and wait for something to jump out at you and if it fails to do so to call it 'normal'. On the contrary you must have a very clear idea in your head of what you are after and ask yourself again and again if it is there. If you do find something wrong you must not fall back in your seat but redouble your efforts and continue ruthlessly with the systematic analysis of the film.

Detecting abnormalities on X-rays can be immensely satisfying. You have in effect got to be like a policeman on the beat, looking for villains, so keep your eyes open and your brain switched on. The stakes are high, but so are the rewards of getting it right!

This book will show you how to do it.

James D. Begg
Dundee
1999

Acknowledgements

I wish to express my grateful thanks to Mrs Ann H. Henderson, Senior Radiographer, Royal Victoria Hospital, Dundee, for her unstinting help with the word processing of the manuscript. Thanks are also due to Dr Colin Paterson, Reader in Medicine and Honorary Consultant Physician, Department of Biochemical Medicine, Ninewells Hospital, Dundee, and Dr Fiona Wood, Senior House Officer in Medicine, Royal Victoria Hospital, Dundee, both of whom provided much appreciated objectivity and helpful comments whilst the book was in preparation.

My appreciation also goes to Mrs Margaret Lawson, Mrs Alice Harrison, Mr Brian Ross and Mr Douglas McNeil of Medical Media Services, Ninewells Hospital, Dundee, for their kind help with all of the X-ray photographs.

I acknowledge with thanks the illustration of a sigmoid volvulus (Fig. 3.13) kindly supplied by Dr H.L. McDonald and Dr R.D. Adams, Consultant Radiologists, Eastern General Hospital, Edinburgh.

Last but not least my thanks must go to Mrs Janice Urquhart, Senior Project Editor and Mr Laurence Hunter, Commissioning Editor, both of Harcourt Publishers, who provided ongoing help and encouragement throughout the course of the project.

James D. Begg

Contents

Chapter 1

How to look at an abdominal X-ray

- The initial inspection of any X-ray begins with a technical assessment. Establishment of the name, date, date of birth, age and sex of the patient at the outset is crucial. There are no prizes for making a brilliant diagnosis in the wrong patient! Further information relating to the ward number or hospital of origin may give an idea as to the potential nature of the patient's problem, e.g. gastrointestinal or urinary, all of which information may be visible on the name badge, so never fail to look at it critically. This can be very helpful in exams. You will notice, however, that the data on the patients' name badges in this book have had to be removed to preserve their anonymity.

- Establish the projection of the film, Virtually every abdominal X-ray is an AP film, i.e. the beam passes from front to back with the film behind the patient, who is lying down with the X-ray machine overhead, but these are frequently accompanied by erect or even decubitus views (also APs). Usually the radiographer will mark the film with a badge or write on it by hand 'Supine' or 'Erect' to guide you, so seek this out and use it.

- Later on you must **learn** to work out for yourself how a given film was taken, from the relative positions of organs, fluid, gas etc.

NB the standard 35×43 cm cassette used to X-ray an adult is tantalisingly smaller than the average normal human abdomen, and usually two films are required to get the entire anatomy included from the diaphragm to the groins. Make sure this has been done before accepting any films for diagnosis. If you don't, you will miss something important and you won't know you've done it! In obese patients cassettes may have to be used transversely, i.e. in 'landscape' as opposed to 'portrait' mode. Rotation is not usually a problem as most patients are happy to lie on their backs.

Underpenetration is not usually such a problem as in the chest. If you can see the bones in the spine, then most of everything else you need to see will probably be visible as well. However, any overexposed (i.e. excessively dark) areas on an X-ray must be inspected again with a bright light behind them (built into many viewing boxes for this purpose, or available as a separate device), as failure to do so may cause you to miss something very important, such as free air under the diaphragm, representing a potentially fatal condition.

It is worth knowing that only five basic densities are normally present on X-rays, which appear thus:

Gas	black
Fat	dark grey
Soft tissue/fluid	light grey
Bone/calcification	white
Metal	intense white

so you can tell from its density what something is made of. There is, however, a summation effect with large organs such as the liver which, because of their bulk, can approach a bony density.

In the abdomen the primary structures outlined are the solid organs, such as the liver, kidneys and spleen; the hollow organs (i.e. the gastrointestinal tract); and the bones. These structures can be classified as:

1. Visible or not visible, and therefore whether present or potentially absent;
2. Too large or too small;
3. Distorted or displaced;
4. Abnormally calcified;
5. Containing abnormal gas, fluid or discrete calculi.

- Take a systematic approach and work your way logically through each group of structures as a checklist. Initial inspection may reveal one or two major and obvious abnormalities, but you must still drill yourself to look through the rest of the film – and you will frequently be surprised by what you find.
- Think logically. You should be able to integrate your knowledge of anatomy, radiographic density and pathology with the findings on the X-ray, and work out what things are and what is going on.
- Look upon X-rays as an extension of physical examination, and regard radiological signs as the equivalent of physical signs in clinical medicine.

- Remember that the X-ray is only a snapshot of the patient at a particular moment in time, and that serious disease may well be present despite a normal initial X-ray. Follow-up films may add the dimension of time and further elucidate the diagnosis, as the radiological signs evolve.

- Remember that however good you are at looking at X-rays there is always someone better at it than you! Never be too embarrassed to show them to a more senior colleague, and always get them reported by a radiologist. He or she is trained to see and extract the maximum amount of useful information from every film, and can frequently help to optimize the care of your patients.

- Remember to provide the radiologist with clear, full, legible and accurate clinical information. This is worth its weight in gold, and will greatly enhance the quality of care of your patients by enhancing the diagnostic value of the films you have requested.

- Finally, a word of caution. In any female of reproductive age check from the LMP (last menstrual period) that she is not pregnant before requesting abdominal X-rays and subjecting her to ionizing radiation. If in doubt and it is not an emergency, discuss it with the radiologist, delay the investigation, or use ultrasound to investigate the problem. If you sign a request form it is your responsibility if you cause a pregnant woman to be X-rayed, and for that you may be sued.

The supine AP film

This is the film most frequently taken and shows most of the structures to the best advantage. The optimum information can only be obtained from it by using the correct viewing conditions. An X-ray should only ever be seriously inspected by uniform transmitted light coming through it, i.e. a viewing box. There is no place for waving it about in the wind as irregular illumination and reflections will prevent 10–20% of the useful information on it being visualized.

Look for (Fig. 1.1):

- The bones of the spine, pelvis, chest cage (ribs) and the sacro-iliac joints
- The dark margins outlining the liver, spleen, kidneys, bladder and psoas muscles – this is intra-abdominal fat
- Gas in the body of the stomach
- Gas in the descending colon
- The wide pelvis, indicating that the patient is female
- Pelvic phleboliths – normal finding
- Minor joint space narrowing in the hips (normal for this age)
- The granular texture of the amorphous fluid faecal matter containing pockets of gas in the caecum, overlying the right iliac bone
- The 'R' marked low down on the right side. The marker can be anywhere on the film and you often have to search for it. All references to 'right' and 'left' refer to the *patient's* right and left. Note the name badge at the bottom, not the top.
- Check that the 'R' marker is compatible with the visible anatomy, e.g.
  – liver on the right
  – left kidney higher than the right
  – stomach on the left
  – spleen on the left
  – heart on the left, when visible.
- The dark skinfold going right across the upper abdomen (normal).

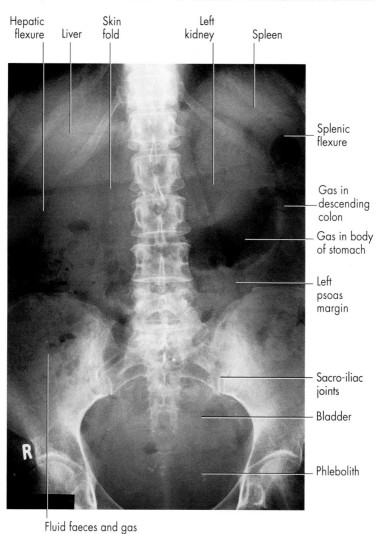

Hepatic flexure

Liver

Skin fold

Left kidney

Spleen

Splenic flexure

Gas in descending colon

Gas in body of stomach

Left psoas margin

Sacro-iliac joints

Bladder

Phlebolith

R

Fluid faeces and gas in caecum

Fig. 1.1 – Adult supine AP radiograph in a 55-year- old woman.

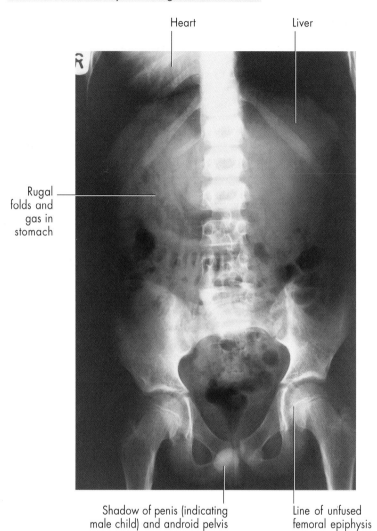

Heart

Liver

Rugal
folds and
gas in
stomach

Shadow of penis (indicating
male child) and android pelvis

Line of unfused
femoral epiphysis

Fig. 1.2 – Supine AP radiograph of a child with left-sided abdominal pain.

Look at (Fig. 1.2):

- The 'right' marker at the top left-hand corner of the film
- The heart shadow on the same side above the right hemidiaphragm (dextro-cardia)
- The outline of the stomach gas and rugal folds on the *right*
- The liver on the *left*
- Unfused epiphyses in the femora. This is a child whose growth is incomplete, his small size leading to the inclusion of the lower chest and upper thighs as well as all of the abdomen – representing a partial 'babygram' as it is known in radiology.

NB This was *not* a radiographic error but a genuine situs inversus with *left-sided appendicitis*.

As with the chest or a limb, establishment of left and right is essential. You do not want to remove a normal kidney from the right side when it is the one on the left that is diseased, because of a faulty X-ray (and this has been done!). Both in exams and in clinical practice situs inversus, or mirror transposition of the abdominal contents, may only be diagnosable from the apparent incompatibility of the L/R marker and the visible anatomy when it has been overlooked clinically.

The L/R marker may of course be incorrectly placed itself as a result of radio-graphic error, and this happens with disturbing frequency (especially with limbs in casualty). You must then go back and check with the radiographer first before misdiagnosing situs inversus, or unnecessarily requesting a further X-ray, as a faulty film can be corrected with a pen. If in doubt, re-examine the patient.

Moral: Always check left and right on every film, consciously and routinely – especially just before surgical operations.

Look at the bones

These provide a useful starting point with which most students are familiar, and are relatively constant in appearance. The lowermost ribs, lumbar spine, sacrum, pelvis and hips are all usually visible to a greater or lesser degree.

The shape of the pelvis will indicate the sex of the patient. The bones may also show evidence of secondary malignant disease, cortical thinning may reflect osteoporosis, and degenerative changes will increase with the age of the patient.

Overlying gas can be a problem in the abdomen, obscuring genuine bone lesions and generating false ones (especially over the sacrum).

The discovery of Paget's disease, myeloma or metastatic disease, however, will often make your search worthwhile.

Look at (Fig. 1.3):

- The bones: the initial routine inspection of the bones showed an incidental finding of extensive sclerosis in the right side of the pelvis compared with the other normal side, and some slight bony expansion.

This is Paget's disease, a premalignant condition in 1% of patients.

Moral: Always check the bones.

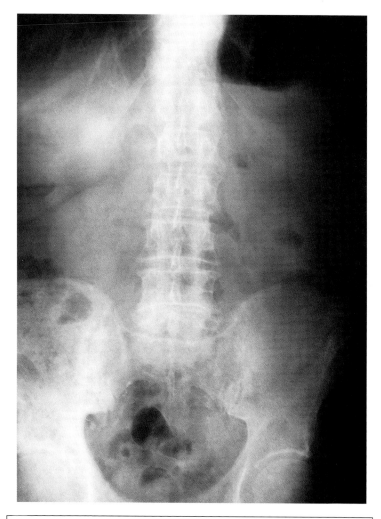

*Fig. 1.3 – **Unilateral sclerosis – right hemipelvis** This is a 62-year-old male patient X-rayed for unexplained abodominal pain. No radiological cause was found on the plain films but endoscopy showed a duodenal ulcer.*

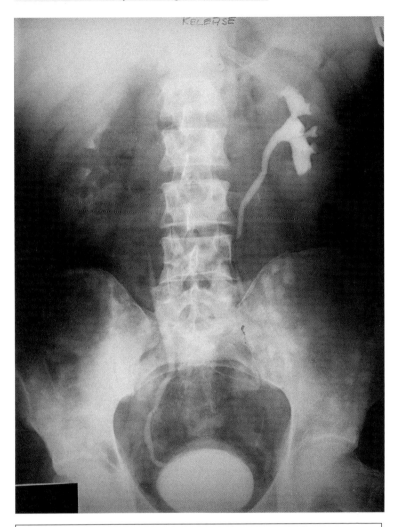

Fig. 1.4 This is a 20-minute IVU film from a 68-year-old man with a craggy mass palpable anteriorly on PR and haematuria.

Look at (Fig. 1.4):

- The bones: there are multiple dense foci in the pelvis and vertebrae of the lumbar spine.

These are typical sclerotic metastases from a carcinoma of the prostate.

Moral: Always check the bones.

Look at (Fig. 1.5):

- The extensive dark material surrounding and starkly contrasting with the gut and especially the kidneys, psoas muscles, liver and spleen.

This is the intraperitoneal and retroperitoneal fat and it is *this* that renders the kidneys and psoas muscles visible on conventional X-ray films. Conversely, replacement of this fat by, for example, haemorrhage or tumour, will obscure these margins.

NB The more fat that is present, the further the kidneys tend to be located away from the spine. This should not be misinterpreted as pathological displacement.

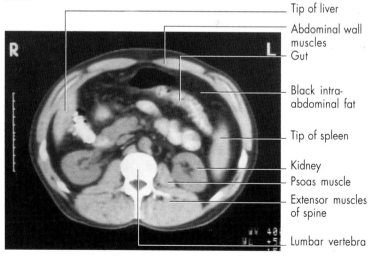

Fig. 1.5 **Intra-abdominal fat** *This is a normal abdominal CT scan at the level of the kidneys.*

11

Look for the psoas muscles (Fig.1.1)

These form two of the few straight lines seen in the body. They form diverging and expanding interfaces extending inferolaterally from the lumbar spine to insert on the lesser trochanters of the femora, and are very important retroperitoneal landmarks. Their non-visualization may reflect serious disease, but there are many benign reasons why they may not be visible, such as an excess of overlying gas, curvature of the spine or a lack of surrounding fat. Always look hard for them but interpret their absence with caution.

Look for the kidneys (Fig. 1.1)

These are usually seen as bean-shaped objects of soft-tissue density high in the upper part of the abdomen. They are usually smooth in outline, extending from the upper border of T12 on the left side to the lower border of L3 on the right side, with the left kidney lying slightly higher than the right and about 1.5 cm bigger. Both kidneys incline slightly medially about 12° towards the spine at their upper poles. Normally they are very mobile, moving down with inspiration, and dropping several centimetres in the erect position. A conscious effort must always be made to find them. Usually, however, only parts of their outlines are visible and you may have to look very hard to try and deduce exactly where they lie and how big they actually are. Occasionally the kidneys may normally be lobulated in outline. This 'fetal lobulation' may then pose diagnostic problems.

Look for the liver (Fig. 1.1)

The liver, being a solid organ in the right upper quadrant, presents as a large area of soft-tissue density, its bulk usually preventing any bowel from occupying this area. Therefore, anywhere that bowel is not present in the right upper quadrant is likely to represent the liver. On occasions, however, bowel can get above the liver and simulate a perforation, i.e. 'Chilaiditi's syndrome', or colonic interposition.

Occasionally an anatomically large extension of the right lobe may occur, looking like a shark's fin, down into the right flank or iliac fossa (a Riedel's lobe). This may well be palpable clinically, but is not a true abnormality. Chronic obstructive pulmonary disease may push the diaphragm and liver down, creating spurious hepatomegaly. Note basal lung markings are often visible through the liver.

Look for the spleen (Fig. 1.1)

This forms a soft tissue mass in the left upper quadrant about the size of the patient's fist or heart. It may be seen well or partially obscured, but in fact is often not seen at all.

Considerable enlargement is necessary to detect it clinically (e.g. up to three times normal), although smaller degrees of enlargement may be shown on a radiograph under favourable conditions. Splenic enlargement greater than 15 cm will tend to displace adjacent structures and has many causes.

Look for the bladder (Fig. 1.1)

Within the pelvis a large mass of soft-tissue density (radiographically water density = soft-tissue density) may be present as a result of a full bladder outlined by perivesical fat, and in females, even normally, volumes up to two litres may occur, pushing all the gut up and out of the true pelvis. If there is doubt as to the nature of such a mass a post-micturition film may be taken or an ultrasound scan done. Being full of fluid, the bladder behaves radiographically like a solid organ.

Look for the uterus

This radiographically solid structure sits on top of and may indent the bladder. It may occasionally be seen spontaneously and is often well demonstrated indirectly at an IVU examination, causing a distinct concavity on the upper edge of the bladder. In many patients, however, it cannot be identified on plain films.

On a normal film, any structure outlined by gas in the abdomen will be part of the gastrointestinal tract. Remember: on a supine AP radiograph the patient is lying on his back, so under gravity any fluid will lie posteriorly within the gut and the gas in the bowel will float anteriorly on top of it.

NB Fluid levels do not appear on supine AP films.

Failure to appreciate this may lead to gross misunderstanding and errors in diagnosis. To demonstrate fluid levels you need an *erect* film or a *decubitus* film taken with a horizontal beam. Think systematically and work your way down through the gastrointestinal tract, identifying structures from the stomach to the rectum.

Look for the stomach

In the supine position, depending on how much is present, the gas in the stomach will rise anteriorly to outline variable volumes of the body and antrum of this structure, to the left of and across the spine around the lowermost thoracic or upper lumbar levels. Simultaneously the resting gastric fluid will form a pool in the fundus beneath the diaphragm, posteriorly on the left-hand side, creating a circular outline – the 'gastric pseudotumour' – which should not be mistaken for an abnormal renal, adrenal or splenic mass, although occasionally it is and requests are received in X-ray to 'investigate the left upper quadrant mass'. Try to avoid this mistake. The mass can be made to disappear by turning the patient prone or sitting him upright, when the familiar fundal gas bubble, commonly best seen on chest X-rays, will appear with a fluid level directly beneath the medial aspect of the left hemidiaphragm (erect film).

Look at (Fig. 1.6):

- The gas lying anteriorly in the body of the stomach
- The fluid pool posteriorly – the gastric pseudotumour.

Gastric pseudotumour in
fundus of stomach

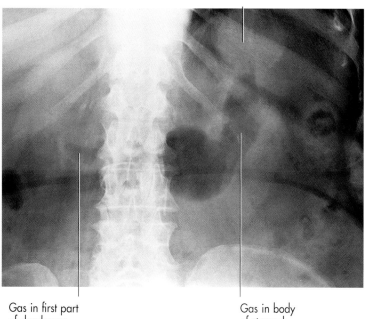

Gas in first part
of duodenum

Gas in body
of stomach

Fig. 1.6 – This is the supine radiograph of an adult, outlining the stomach.

Look at (Fig. 1.7):

- How the barium pools in the fundus, exactly as the resting gastric juice does on the plain film
- The large amount of gas present, again in the body of the stomach. The patient has in fact been given effervescent powder to generate excess carbon dioxide to distend the stomach and generate 'double contrast', i.e. an outline of the mucosa with barium and gas .
- How the fundus is seen only in 'single contrast' on this view, i.e. barium alone.

Look for the small bowel

Because of peristalsis the outline of the gas in the normal small bowel is often broken up into many small pockets which form polygonal shapes, but occupy a generally central location in the abdomen. When more distended, the characteristic 'valvulae conniventes', or coiled spring-shaped folds, crossing the entire lumen may be seen in the jejunum, although the normal ileum tends to remain featureless. The calibre of the normal small bowel should not exceed 2.5cm–3cm, increasing slightly distally.

Often very little is seen of the small bowel on plain films, as in Figure 1.1, and it only becomes well visualised when abnormal.

Barium pooling in fundus

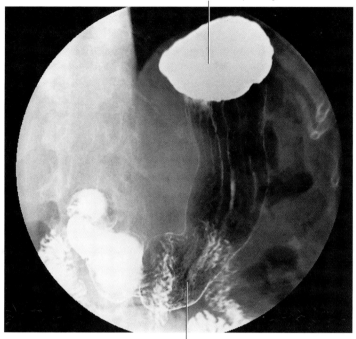

Gas in body of stomach

Fig. 1.7 – This is a spot film from a barium meal study with the patient supine – exactly the same position as the preceding film.

Look for the appendix

You'll be lucky to find it! Occasionally this structure will contain an 'appendicolith' (i.e. calcified faecal material) which may predispose the patient to appendicitis Less commonly gas will be present in the appendix, sometimes barium from a recent GI study, or even pieces of lead shot which have been ingested and impacted themselves there.

If you see this (Fig. 1.8) you can then have a little bit of amusement with your patients, who will be amazed to know how you have figured out from their abdominal X-ray that they have recently eaten game (e.g. a rabbit or a pheasant).

Note: Retained barium in the appendix implies the previous administration of barium, either, orally or per rectum, and implies suspected GI tract disease. If barium enters the appendix, however, it implies that this organ is normal.

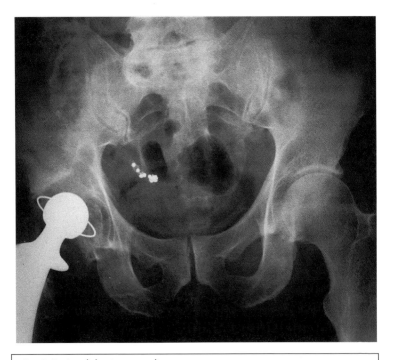

Fig. 1.8 – Lead shot in appendix

Look for the colon (Figs 1.1 and 1.9)

1. Start with the caecum in the right iliac fossa. The caecum is the most distensible part of the colon and receives fluid material directly from the ileum through the ileocaecal valve. The caecum therefore normally contains semifluid material containing multiple pockets of gas and, like much of the right side of the bowel, assumes a granular appearance on X-rays, creating mottled areas of gas seen best against the background of the iliac bone. On occasions the normal caecum may be empty.

2. **NB** The classic anatomical layout of the colon is often found to be deviated from by tortuous and redundant bowel, but the hepatic and splenic flexures should be identifiable as the highest fixed points on the right and left sides, respectively. The transverse colon may dip down deeply into the pelvis, but the faecal content of the bowel becomes increasingly solid and formed as one passes distally, eventually generating discrete masses which may be individually identified, but which always contain many tiny pockets of gas.

3. Learn to identify faecal material on abdominal X-rays (see Fig. 3.10). Find *that* and you've found the *colon*, which may be very important in film analysis, particularly in differentiating small bowel from large bowel. These findings can best be appreciated in severe constipation with gross faecal overload. Sometimes this will involve the rectum (which is usually empty in normal individuals), when a large faecal plug may be present associated with overflow incontinence.

4. When visible the haustral folds of the colon may be seen, only partially visualized across part of the large bowel lumen, although in some patients complete crossing of the lumen by haustra may occur.

Under the effects of gravity much changes when an abdominal X-ray is taken in the **erect** position. The major events are:

- Air rises
- Fluid sinks
- Kidneys drop
- Transverse colon drops
- Small bowel drops
- Breasts drop (females: they lie laterally when supine)
- Lower abdomen bulges and increases in X-ray density
- Diaphragm descends causing increased clarity of lung bases.

The liver and spleen, being fixed, tend to become more visible, the remaining mid and lower abdominal contents less so. When the lower abdomen bulges under gravity this reduces the clarity of its contents owing to the crowding together of organs and the consequent increased density of the soft tissues. Depending on the original height of the colon and their own descent in the erect position, the kidneys may become more or less visible.

The erect film, however, may now show **fluid levels** (see Fig. 3.4), which can be very helpful in confirming the diagnosis of obstruction and abscesses, but fluid levels on normal films tend to be very small or invisible. In perforation of the bowel an erect film may confirm a pneumoperitoneum, when gas has risen to the classic subdiaphragmatic position.

Look at (Fig. 1.9 — NB that this is a different patient from Fig. 1.1):

- The 'ERECT' marker over T11
- The dependent position of the breasts, causing increased densities over the right and left upper quadrants. Do not mistake these for the liver or spleen – their edges pass laterally beyond the confines of the abdomen
- The gas in the gastric fundus – typical of the erect position
- Small quantities of trapped gas between and outlining the gastric rugal folds in this patient
- The film is centred high, showing the lung bases but missing part of the pelvis
- The position of the colon, which has dropped under gravity, and bulging of the lower abdomen anteriorly, causing the increased density in the lower third of the abdomen and obscuring the anatomy.

Gas in fundus of stomach

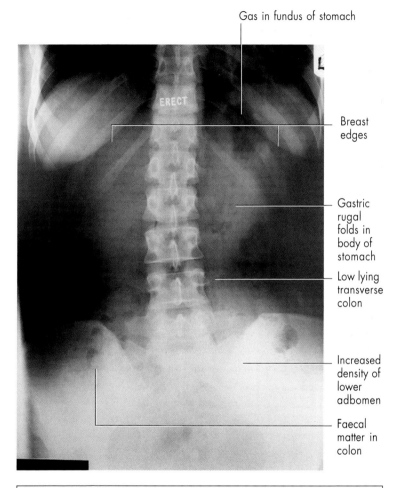

Breast edges

Gastric rugal folds in body of stomach

Low lying transverse colon

Increased density of lower adbomen

Faecal matter in colon

Fig. 1.9 – This is a typical normal erect abdominal radiograph of a female patient but there is insufficient fluid to form fluid levels.

Look for normal calcified structures

Learn to recognize the following structures, which can normally calcify and cause diagnostic confusion:

Costal cartilages may be mistaken for ..... Biliary and renal calculi
Hepatic and splenic calcification
Old TB in lung bases

Aorta may be mistaken for .... Aortic aneurysm (if tortuous or bent)

Iliac arteries may be mistaken for .... Iliac aneurysms (if tortuous or bent)

Splenic artery, 'The Chinese
dragon sign', may be mistaken for .... Splenic artery aneurysms

Pelvic phleboliths may be mistaken for .. Ureteric/bladder calculi

Mesenteric lymph nodes may be
mistaken for .... Renal/ureteric calculi/sclerotic bone
lesions over spine/sacrum/ilium.

Red faces all round and serious consequences for the patient from misdiagnosis may occur from misinterpreting these normal findings. Don't let it happen to *you!*

Costal cartilages

On abdominal and chest X-rays look at the rib ends. In many patients they often appear to stop suddenly and nothing is seen of the costal cartilages. Keep looking, however, and in others a continuation of the ribs will clearly be seen. This can be marginal, heavy and distinctive in males, or more punctate and central in females, and the phenomenon increases with age, but occasionally can be startlingly heavy in the young.

Look at (Fig. 1.10):

- The multiple dense foci over the upper and middle abdomen. This is costal cartilage calcification, which both simulates and can obscure genuine associated areas of calcification in the underlying organs, such as TB or calculi in the liver, kidneys or spleen.

What to do? Oblique films, tomograms or CT scanning may be required for further elucidation or the exclusion of calculi. Tomograms are X-ray films which select out slices at different levels and blur the backgrounds.

Artefact   Costal cartilage calcification

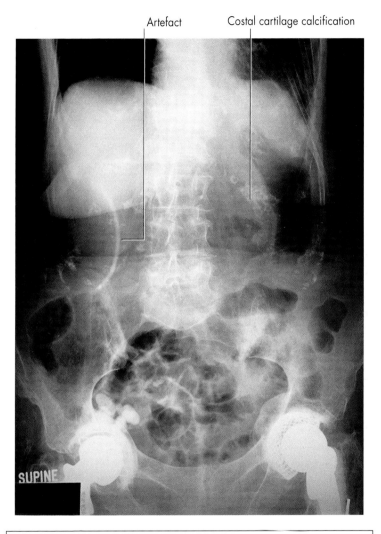

SUPINE

Fig. 1.10 – AP radiograph of a 75-year-old woman.

Aorta

Look at (Fig. 1.11):

- The calcified aorta over the lumbar spine, dividing at the inferior body of L4 into the iliac arteries, which cross L5 and both sacral wings. You will often also see interrupted linear calcification in both walls of the common and external iliac arteries, which may continue across the true pelvis to the femoral arteries in the groins, representing arteriosclerotic changes.
- With increasing age the aorta shows increased calcification, just like the aortic knuckle in the chest, and starts to become visible over the age of 40. Look carefully over the lumbar spine area for flecks of parallel or slightly converging plaques of calcification which may be seen: **you must train yourself to look for this routinely on every film in order to exclude an aneurysm.** Be careful, however, not to mistake a curving osteophyte in an osteoarthritic spine for the aorta or an aneurysm.
- In some patients the aorta can become tortuous and bent to the left or the right of the spine, but without becoming aneurysmal.
- Look at **both** calcified walls for loss of **parallelism** before diagnosing an aneurysm, as simple tortuous vessels and aneurysms can look like each other.
- Note the **age** of every patient carefully. Premature calcification in the aorta can be a very significant medical finding – e.g. in diabetes or chronic renal failure – and is not always due to physiological changes of ageing.

Calcified aorta

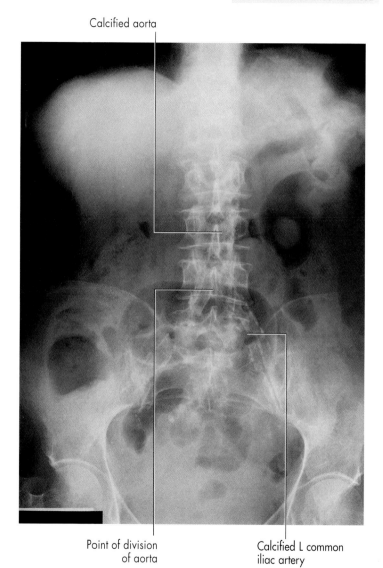

Point of division
of aorta

Calcified L common
iliac artery

Fig. 1.11 – Supine AP radiograph of a 68-year-old woman.

Pelvic phleboliths

Look at (Fig. 1.12):

The true pelvis. There are small round smooth opacities, some of which contain lucent centres. These are phleboliths. There may be just one or two of these 'vein stones' (literal translation from the Greek) or a great number of them. In themselves they are usually without clinical significance, but they may require exclusion as ureteric calculi by an IVU in patients who present with renal colic, and not every pelvic opacity is by any means a urinary tract stone. Rarely they may be part of a pelvic haemangioma.

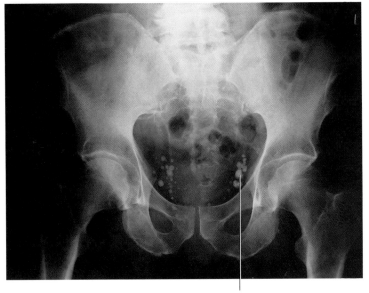

Phleboliths

Fig. 1.12 – AP view of the pelvis in a 53-year-old woman.

Look at (Fig. 1.13):

- The small opacity in the L true pelvis: phlebolith or calculus?

A control film (p. 28) has several purposes:

- To try to locate the position of the kidneys before injection
- To look for calculi
- To exclude an aortic aneurysm – compression by a tight belt is often applied across the lower abdomen during IVUs, but not in renal colic, other acute abdomens, postoperative states or trauma. The purpose is to prevent inadvertent compression of an aneurysm
- To demonstrate any incidental findings
- To check the radiographic and processing quality prior to the contrast injection and taking of further films
- To look for evidence of metastases in suspected malignancy.

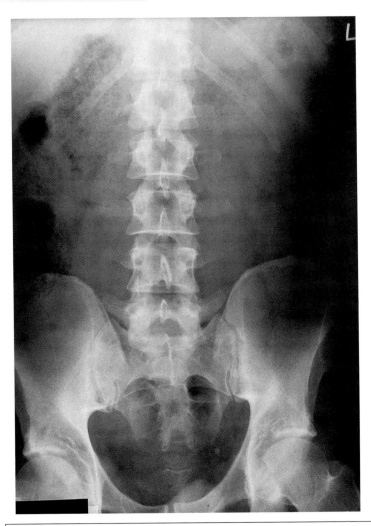

Fig. 1.13 – This is the supine AP radiograph of a 45-year-old male who presented with suspected L renal colic. Urologists refer to such radiographs as 'KUB' films, for Kidneys, Ureters and Bladder. Other names include 'SCOUT' films and 'PRELIM' films, but the correct radiogical term is a 'CONTROL' film. This means an X-ray taken to assess the patient before any contrast medium has been given.

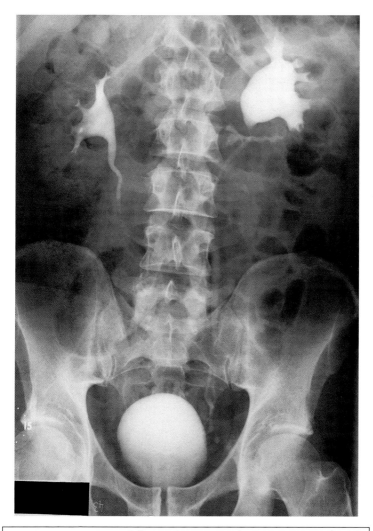

Fig. 1.14 – Same patient following the injection of contrast. Note how the left ureter has bypassed the pelvic opacity, which is now shown not to be a calculus but a phlebolith. The cause of the patient's pain was at a much higher level, i.e. the left pelviureteric junction, which is narrowed and causing dilatation (hydronephrosis) of the left renal pelvis.

Splenic artery

The splenic artery may only be intermittently calcified, the discontinuity making it more difficult to identify its true nature than in Figure 1.15. Partial splenic arterial calcification must not be misinterpreted as a splenic artery aneurysm.

Do not mistake it for renal artery calcification: this may of course coexist and will often be present bilaterally, but usually only the splenic artery shows such a degree of tortuosity as it wends its way towards the splenic hilum. Heavy overlying costal cartilage calcification (Fig. 1.15) may make it difficult to isolate the splenic arterial calcification.

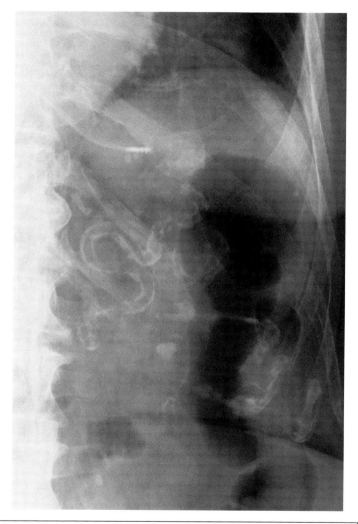

Fig. 1.15 – **Calcified splenic artery** This is the left upper quadrant of a 78-year-old woman. Note the serpiginous parallel-walled calcified lesion in the left flank, resembling a 'jumping jack' firework or 'Chinese dragon' extending towards the hilum of the spleen. This is the splenic artery.

Calcified lymph nodes

Look at (Fig. 1.16):

- The incidental finding of a collection of granular opacities in the flanks
- The partially coalescent cluster of opacities over the L3/4/5 lumbar spine levels
- Some further small opacities in the epigastrium.

These are calcified lymph nodes. Usually the patient is asymptomatic in regard to these. Lying in the mesentery they tend to be quite mobile and show dramatic changes in position from film to film. Conversely, an apparently sclerotic lesion in a lumbar vertebra can be shown by an erect or slightly rotated oblique film to be mobile and due to an overlying calcified lymph node. Always remember that on an X-ray you are looking at three-dimensional structures lying on top of each other shown in only two dimensions. Calcified mesenteric lymph nodes are often attributed to previous ingestion of TB bacilli to the gut, which have been halted at the regional lymph nodes. On occasion they will require to be excluded a renal or ureteric calculi, and can be a real diagnostic nuisance.

NB Calcified *retroperitoneal* lymph nodes, or such nodes opacified by contrast medium at lymphography, may also overlie the spine but show less relative motion, being very posterior. Calcified nodes require to be differentiated from calculi and calcification in underlying organs right alongside the spine or iliac vessels.

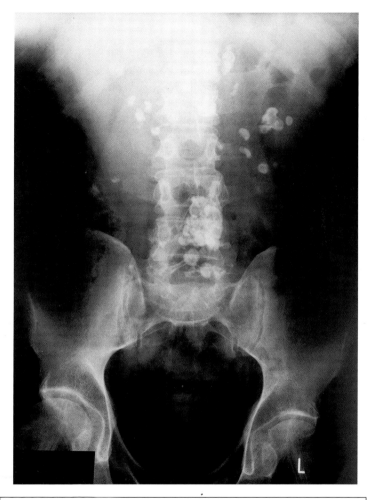

Fig. 1.16 – This is a supine AP abdominal radiograph of a 45-year-old male X-rayed for abdominal pain.

A word about decubitus films (Fig. 3.9)

- The Latin word *decubitus* comes from the Latin *decumbere:* 'to lie down', like a Roman patrician lying on his side eating at a banquet, and means with the patient lying on his left or right side. Its purpose is to obtain further information, such as confirmation of a small amount of free gas, or to demonstrate fluid levels in a patient too ill to be sat up. A horizontal cross-table beam is used rather than the usual vertical beam from overhead for supine films.

- Such films require very close and careful interpretation and should not be taken blindly without a very clear idea of what is being sought, usually in conjunction with the radiologist, or as a reasonable alternative to an erect view for the radiographer. Such films, however, may be very valuable and clinch the diagnosis – if 5 or 10 minutes are spent with the patient in the appropriate position to allow any free gas to track up to the flank. If you take it too early you may miss the gas, as the amount is sometimes very small.

- Decubitus films can be identified by fluid levels lying parallel to the long axis of the body, as opposed to at right-angles to it on conventional erect films (see film of the scrotum on p. 71). They are also used routinely during conventional barium enema examinations, and to demonstrate free pleural fluid in the chest, e.g. to differentiate a 'subpulmonary' effusion from a raised hemidiaphragm, and to optimize the view of the uppermost lung bases in patients who cannot inspire fully.

NB A 'right decubitus' means the patient is lying with his right side down. A 'left decubitus' means the patient is lying with his left side down.

For technical reasons decubitus films tend to come out very dark (i.e. over exposed) and frequently require bright lights behind them to allow them to be studied properly.

They are best shared with, and interpreted by the radiologist *at the time they are taken*. Getting a report of a perforation (which you have missed) the next day when the patient is dead is too late.

Chapter 2

Solid organs

Big liver

- Like feet and noses, livers come in different shapes and sizes. Just as a liver may appear to be significantly enlarged clinically by palpation, it may also look enlarged on an abdominal X-ray when in fact neither is the case, and such assessment is often subjective.

- As already mentioned, livers pushed down by lungs chronically overinflated by chronic obstructive pulmonary disease, or having an anatomically more extensive right lobe (see Fig 6.19), can both create this illusion, and these facts must be remembered. Conversely, true hepatomegaly must be suspected when there is evidence of displacement of adjacent organs or, as a rough guide, when the length of the liver exceeds around 16 cm from the apex of the right hemidiaphragm in the parasagittal plane, but clinical and radiological findings may not concur.

- Liver enlargement is of course a very non-specific sign, and serves only as a reason for launching further investigations of both liver function and imaging – usually ultrasound to begin with.

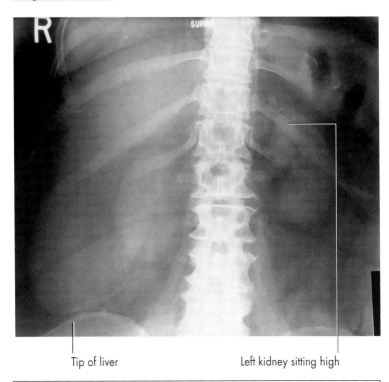

Tip of liver   Left kidney sitting high

Fig. 2.1 – Abdominal radiograph of a 68-year-old woman with a large palpable mass in the R side of the abdomen.

Look at (Fig. 2.1):

- The huge mass in the R side of the abdomen reaching to the level of the iliac crest
- The absence of gut in the R side of the abdomen which has been displaced
- The increased density of the R side of the abdomen
- The rounded configuration of the lower edge of the mass
- The entire margin of the normal R kidney remaining clearly preserved by its surrounding fat, indicating that the mass is not renal
- The R marker confirming this is consistent with the liver
- The left kidney sitting high (upper margin T11).

This is gross hepatomegaly. Occasionally elevation of the R hemidiaphragm or downward displacement of the R kidney are other signs to look for on chest and abdominal films. The high left kidney causes spurious apparent downward displacement of the left one.

Point to ponder: in children the normal liver takes up a disproportionate amount of space compared with the adult.

Liver enlargement

The main causes are:

Malignant	Metastases, hepatoma, cholangiocarcinoma
Metabolic storage diseases	Glycogen, amyloid, fat
Inflammatory	Hepatitis, abscesses, parasites etc.
Cirrhosis	Early stages
Vascular	Heart failure, pericarditis
Haematological	Myelofibrosis, leukaemia

Small liver

The liver may look to be on the small side and yet be normal anatomically and functionally, e.g. in a small individual, and declaring a liver to be pathologically shrunken from a plain abdominal X-ray is not normally attempted.

A secondary effect of shrinkage of the liver, however, may be that a loop of colon – or, less frequently, small bowel – may slip above it and become visible directly beneath the right hemidiaphragm (see Colonic interposition, Fig. 4.5). The appearance of such a loop does not, however, prove that the liver has reduced in size, as this phenomenon may occur in an otherwise normal individual. It is also more likely to be seen in patients with large thoracic outlets (COPD), or postoperatively when the surgeon has pushed the viscera aside to get at something else.

The usual cause for shrinkage of the liver is the late stage of cirrhosis, this itself having a number of causes, e.g.:

- Alcohol
- Hepatitis
- Drugs
- Obstruction.

Coexisting enlargement of the spleen may occur, with associated portal hypertension.

Big spleen

Frequently the spleen cannot be seen on an abdominal X-ray. When enlarged (>15cm), as with other intra-abdominal masses, this is detected by an increase in size and density, and by displacement of adjacent structures. A normal spleen can indent the left kidney, causing a 'splenic hump' just below the point of contact (which must not be mistaken for a true renal swelling), and small accessory spleens can sometimes be present.

NB Occasionally a patient will have no spleen, due either to congenital absence or surgical removal.

Splenomegaly can, however, be enormous, especially when the patient comes late to medical attention. This finding, like hepatomegaly, is non-specific and has many causes.

Look for (Fig. 2.2):

- A soft tissue mass extending downwards and medially from the left upper quadrant
- Elevation of the left hemidiaphragm
- Medial displacement of the stomach
- Downward displacement of the left kidney
- Inferior displacement of the colon
- Evidence of associated liver enlargement and lymph node enlargement.

NB Occasionally the spleen will enlarge selectively down the Ⓛ flank lateral to the Ⓛ kidney.

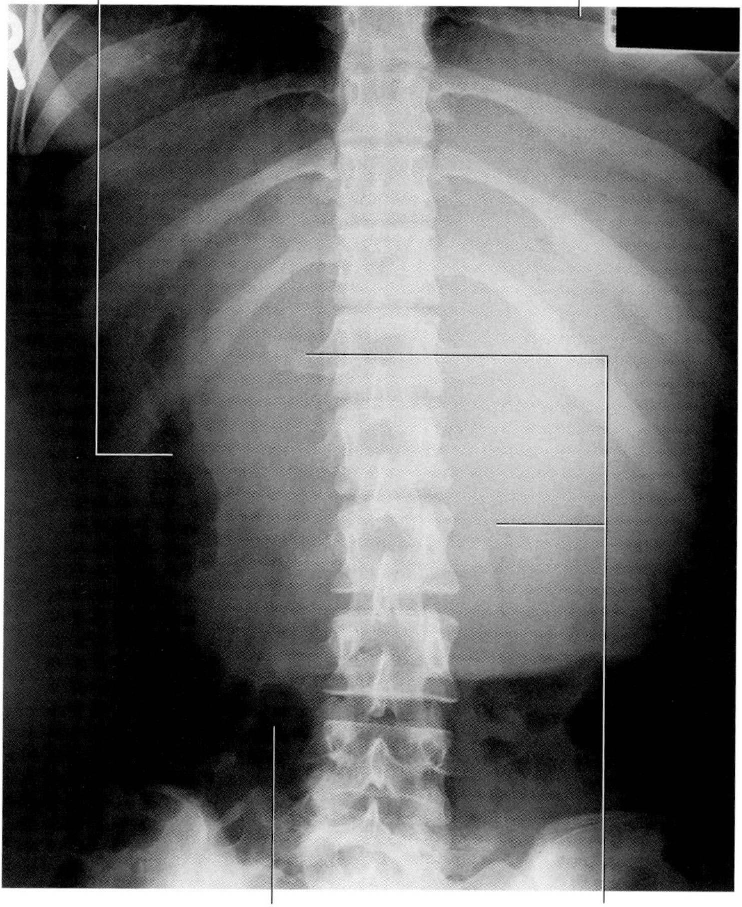

Stomach displaced to
right side of abdomen

Elevated left
hemidiaphragm

Depressed transverse colon

Spleen

*Fig. 2.2 – **Splenomegaly** This is the film of an adult female who presented with generalized ill health and a large mass in the left upper abdomen. Examination of the blood showed changes of leukaemia. The mass was shown on ultrasound to be a large spleen. The liver was not enlarged. Note the R marker just visible at the top left-hand corner of the film.*

Causes of splenomegaly

Trauma	Rupture of spleen, causing apparent splenomegaly from a subcapsular haematoma
Infection	Acute: Infectious mononucleosis
	Infective endocarditis
	Chronic: TB
	Brucellosis
	HIV
	Malaria
Neoplasm	Secondaries from bronchus, breast, gut, prostate
Lymphomatous	Hodgkins' disease
	Non-Hodgkins' disease
Haematological	Leukaemia
	Polycythaemia
	Myelosclerosis
	Haemolytic anaemia
Storage disorders	Gaucher's disease
Portal hypertension	
Cystic masses	Polycystic disease
	Hydatid cyst
	Developmental cysts
Others	Rheumatoid
	Amyloid
	Sarcoid
	Collagen vascular diseases

Big kidneys

Note (Fig. 2.3):

- The bulky but smoothly outlined kidneys
- Normal kidneys extend from approximately the lower margin of T12 on the left to the upper margin of L3 on the right, or about 3.5 vertebral bodies (plus discs)
- These kidneys extend from the upper margin of T12 on the left to the upper margin of L4 on the right, or 4.5 vertebral bodies (and discs) in this patient.

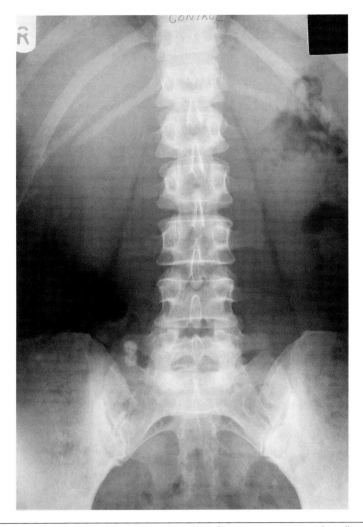

*Fig. 2.3 – **Enlarged kidneys** This is the film of a patient presenting clinically with symptoms and signs of acute glomerulonephritis with fever, blood and protein in the urine.*

- Kidneys vary in size and shape and the left one is usually slightly larger than the right by up to 1.5 cm, although a duplex kidney (i.e. one with a double drainage system) may look abnormally big but still be histologically normal.
- Kidneys are usually larger in men than in women, and each individual kidney should not normally be more than about 3.5 vertebral bodies long, including the intervening lumbar discs in a given patient, measured in their long axes, i.e. from pole to pole inclined towards the spine. Kidneys over 12 cm and under 9 cm are usually regarded as pathologically large and small, respectively. Kidneys in young children normally appear disproportionately large just as the liver does.
- Bilaterally enlarged or unilaterally enlarged kidneys may be present with one normal size or shrunken on the contralateral side. Enlargement of each kidney may also be generalized due to global disease or something more focal, such as a cyst, tumour or localized hypertrophy. So-called compensatory hypertrophy of a remaining kidney may also occur if the other one ceases to function or is removed, but this response reduces in the elderly.
- The importance of detecting large kidneys is that there may be the potential for recovery when this finding is associated with renal failure, although biopsy will be required for definitive diagnosis, almost invariably preceded by ultrasound to help exclude renal obstruction and assess the parenchyma.
- Conversely, small kidneys usually reflect end-stage renal disease and an irreversible state, making biopsy somewhat academic and potentially hazardous.
- Look carefully too at the edges of the kidneys, whether smooth, lobulated or irregular – important points in differential diagnosis.

Causes of bilateral big kidneys

- Acute glomerulonephritis
- Diabetic renal disease (glomerulosclerosis)
- Adult polycystic disease
- Acute tubular necrosis
- Acute cortical necrosis
- Bilateral acute pyelonephritis
- Leukaemic infiltration
- Lymphomatous infiltration

- Amyloid
- Secondary renal disease in gout.
- Excessive beer drinking – medical students please note!

Some causes of unilateral big kidney

- Acute obstruction
- Acute infarction: renal artery occlusion, renal vein thrombosis
- Acute pyelonephritis
- Radiation nephritis
- Duplex system
- Compensatory hypertrophy from contralateral nephrectomy or dysfunction
- Renal mass.

Small kidneys

Establishing the presence of small kidneys may be very difficult or impossible on plain films owing to overlying faeces and gas. However, if the patient is clearly alive and not on dialysis there must be functioning renal tissue somewhere, and occasionally it is visible.

Remember: The kidneys shrink or atrophy with age, compensatory hypertrophy may not occur in the elderly, and X-ray measurements will always give a 20–25% magnification, so that X-ray measurements will always be larger than sizes obtained on ultrasound, CT or MRI examinations, for example; the apparent size of the kidneys may also increase even more after i.v. contrast administration for IVUs.

Causes of small kidneys

- Chronic glomerulosclerosis (usually bilateral)
- Chronic ischaemia (e.g. renal artery stenosis, arteriosclerosis)
- Chronic pyelonephritis
- Reflux nephropathy
- Infarction
- Senile atropy
- Congenital hypoplasia (usually unilateral).

NB **Always remember that an unknown patient may have only one functioning kidney.** This is especially important when investigating trauma: more than one patient in medical history has had his only kidney taken out, and kidneys have a remarkable capacity for healing and regeneration.

NB **A patient who is known to have only one functioning kidney and who is passing urine cannot be completely obstructed.** This is sometimes forgotten by young doctors requesting 'urgent' IVUs for '? obstruction' when one kidney has been removed.

Two important congenital renal abnormalities

Pelvic kidneys

When investigations fail to demonstrate kidneys in the renal beds, one or more of them is usually found at a lower level in the pelvis. This is called an ectopic kidney (Greek *ek*, out of, *topos*, place). Inflamed pelvic kidneys can simulate appendicitis or gynaecological problems. Remember: transplanted kidneys may be put into the pelvis and even a normally sited kidney may be invisible.

Horseshoe kidneys

These can sometimes be suspected or diagnosed on plain films. They tend to lie lower than normal and tend to lack the usual medial inclination relative to the spine at their upper poles. The pathognomonic radiological sign is to see the renal cortices of the lower kidneys crossing the margins of the psoas muscles medially to connect with the other side. This part of a horseshoe kidney system is known as the isthmus. The drainage systems in this condition tend to be malrotated forwards. The isthmus may contain either functioning or just fibrous tissue.

Look at (Fig. 2.4):

- The cortical margins of the kidneys crossing the psoas muscles
- The associated developmental spinal anomaly at the L3/4 level on the left and the scoliosis convex to the left.

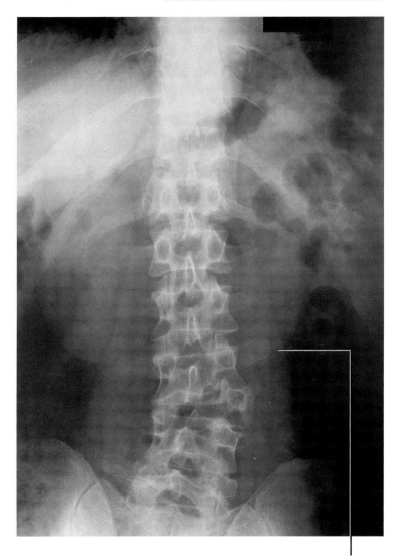

Renal cortex crossing the psoas muscle

Fig. 2.4 – Horse shoe kidneys

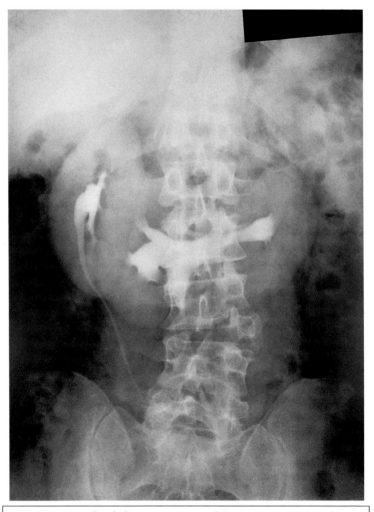

*Fig. 2.5 – **Horseshoe kidneys** Same patient following i.v. contrast confirming horseshoe kidneys.*

Look at (Fig. 2.5):

- The abnormal fused renal collecting systems overlying the spine and the isthmus
- The malrotated right kidney with its collecting system facing antero-laterally instead of medially.

Complications

Horseshoe kidneys are more susceptible to infection, stone formation and trauma.

The isthmus may also get in the way in radiotherapy planning. Horseshoe kidneys may occur in Turner's syndrome.

Renal masses

Renal masses may be found during the investigation of a patient with urinary tract symptoms, such as haematuria, or as an incidental finding when the patient is being X-rayed for some other purpose, e.g. backache, but even a large one may be invisible on a standard film. A significant renal mass may however:

- Distort the position of the anticipated renal outline
- Actually displace the kidney from which it arises
- Displace overlying gas-containing loops of bowel
- Cross the midline to the opposite side.

Having detected a mass the primary requirement is then to establish whether it is solid or cystic, and this can usually be easily achieved with ultrasound. Further careful inspection of the plain films in the initial phase, however, to look for loss of psoas outlines or bony destruction of part of a vertebra, may indicate malignancy from the outset. Looking into the lung bases on an abdominal X-ray may also on occasion reveal pulmonary metastases, and should be routine on all abdominal X-rays where these are visible, although a full chest X-ray will already be indicated.

The next task is staging with CT of the mass, MRI etc.

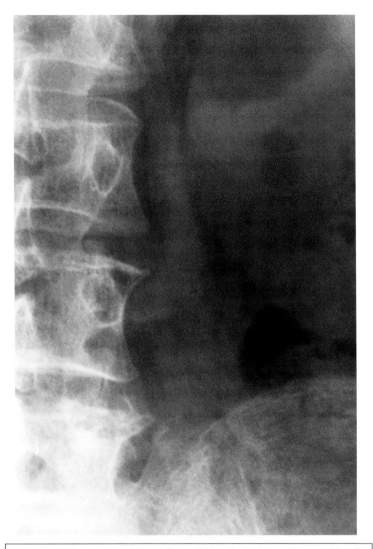

Fig. 2.6 – Close-up view from abdominal film of L flank in a 56-year-old male presenting with backache.

This patient (Fig. 2.6) initially had his lumbar spine and abdomen X-rayed to look for a cause for his backache. Apart from minor degenerative change no skeletal abnormality was found, but careful inspection of the film showed the edge of a large mass in the left flank which was clearly too big to represent part of a normal kidney. An ultrasound scan confirmed a solid mass arising from the left kidney. On biopsy this was found to be a renal carcinoma.

Moral: Do not confine yourself to the area of primary interest alone on an X-ray film, but look at all of it. Always be ready for the unexpected incidental finding.

A word about 'displacing masses'

Obviously an abnormal mass can arise anywhere and its general effect will be the same, i.e. to produce a dense area with displacement of bowel loops around it. Sophisticated investigations will be necessary to establish the exact cause (ultrasound, CT, MRI, barium etc.). Should the mass itself contain a lot of gas this will usually indicate part of the bowel itself (e.g. volvulus) or perhaps an abscess (see Figs 4.13 and 4.14). The density of a mass may also be increased by the presence of calcification within it.

The urinary bladder

In practice the most common reason for finding a large mass on X-ray in the pelvis is a full bladder (Fig. 1.1), and there are a number of reasons for this:

1. Patients often have to wait to be brought to X-ray and their transit may be delayed.
2. Further waiting periods are common in busy X-ray departments.
3. Some patients will have genuine outflow obstruction, e.g. due to prostatic disease, and be unable to empty their bladders completely. Some patients who come back for KUB films and renal ultrasound are specifically asked to attend with a full bladder.

In seeking the bladder, look for:
- A smooth rounded or transversely orientated oval mass of uniform density in the pelvis. Its outline, when visible, is due to perivesical fat (see Fig. 1.1)
- Upward displacement of small bowel loops, which are freely mobile and can easily be shifted completely out of the pelvis
- Excessive indentations in addition to the normal ones (sigmoid and uterus) caused by pathologically enlarged masses (e.g. fibroids) or faecal overload.

Common causes of pelvic masses
- Physiologically full bladder: male or female
- Pathologically full bladder indicating outflow obstruction, e.g. prostate in an adult male or a blocked catheter in a female
- Bulky uterus (pregnancy) – look for fetal parts! Did you check the LMP (last menstrual period) before requesting this film?

The majority of significant abnormal pelvic masses occur in females, including:
- Leiomyomas – fibroids, often calcified
- Ovarian cysts – can be the size of a football
- Ovarian tumours (benign or malignant)
- Pelvic inflammatory disease/abscesses
- Haematometra (blood collection in uterus)
- Endometriosis
- Haematocolpos (blood collection behind imperforate hymen)
- Dermoids, containing fat, teeth, hair.

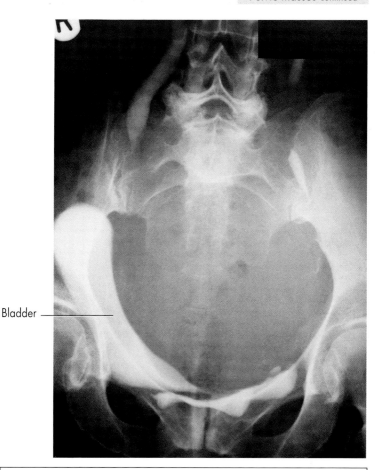

Bladder

Fig. 2.7 – AP pelvis: IVU examination, bladder area. Look at the effect of a huge pelvic mass severely compressing the bladder from above. This was an ovarian cyst. It is also partially obstructing both ureters.

Non-gynaecological

- Abscesses from appendix, diverticula, lymphocoele (postoperatively)
- Pelvic kidney (congenital)
- Renal transplant.

These usually obscure the psoas muscle on the affected side or show a displaced fat line convex and beyond the margins of the anticipated position of the psoas muscle. They may show displacement of the kidneys (see Fig. 2.8) or aorta, are often malignant, e.g. lymphadenopathy, and require further investigation.

Do not mistake slight convexity of the normally straight psoas margins for pathology. These can hypertrophy in very athletic individuals, just like the gastrocnemius muscles. Such individuals may also show incipient degenerative changes in the hips in early adult life and medial deviation of the ureters on an IVU – signs to seek in confirmation.

Look at (Fig. 2.8):

- The absence of the normally positioned psoas edge on the left side and convex mass more lateral to it
- Normal spleen
- Upward and lateral displacement of the left kidney.

This is retroperitoneal lymphadenopathy, due to lymphoma.

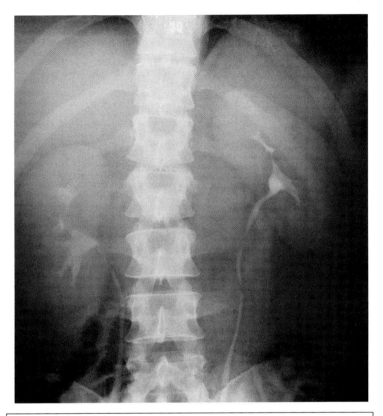

Fig. 2.8 – This is an IVU film showing renal excretion in a young man who presented with a mass in the neck, weight loss and backache.

There are no plain film signs that confirm or exclude acute pancreatitis. The diagnosis is a clinical one supported by high serum amylase levels. Chest and abdominal films will, however, usually have been taken on admission while the diagnosis is being sorted out. Imaging this condition and its complications is a job for ultrasound or CT, but underlying causes and secondary effects may occasionally be identified.

Look for:

- Gallstones (may be a predisposing factor)
- Calcification in the pancreas (chronic pancreatitis may be complicated by recurrent bouts of acute pancreatitis). Occasionally a tumour containing calcification may precipitate pancreatitis
- Pleural effusions, basal atelectasis, diaphragmatic elevation
- Signs of secondary ileus
- Rarely in severe disease gas bubbles may appear in the pancreas as abscess formation supervenes
- Retroperitoneal gas/pneumoperitoneum – rarely and usually in severe disease. May be confused with perforation
- Ascitic fluid
- Bone infarcts e.g. head of femur (very rare).

Chapter 3

Hollow organs

The stomach

Look at (Fig. 3.1):

- Abnormally large size of the gastric outline
- Excessive quantity of semidigested food in the stomach
- Small quantity of gas in the small bowel.

Look at (Fig. 3.2):

- The two fluid levels, that on the left representing the gastric fundus and that on the right the duodenum – the so-called 'double-bubble sign'.
- The actual level of obstruction is in the duodenum, caused by scarring and stenosis from ulcer disease.

NB This sign may also be seen in neonates with duodenal atresia.

Causes of gastric outflow obstruction

- Peptic ulcer disease in distal stomach/duodenum with scarring
- Gastric carcinoma in antrum
- Lymphoma
- Gastritis
- Crohn's disease (stomach or duodenum)
- TB
- Impacted foreign bodies
- Bezoar (furball, vegetable matter)
- Metastases.

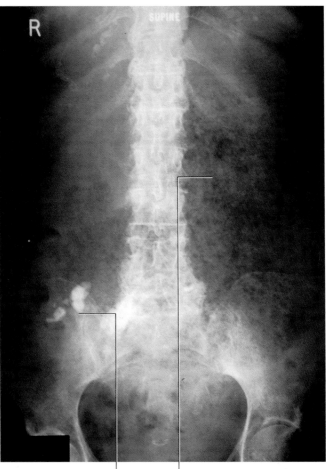

Calcified
lymph nodes

Extensive semi-digested food and gas in
the stomach filling much of the abdomen

Fig. 3.1 – A 54-year-old man with a 2-year history of dyspepsia who presented
with upper abdominal distension, a succussion splash and vomiting. This was
due to outflow obstruction and retention of food residue and fluid. A 'bezoar'
looks similar – retained vegetable matter (phytobezoar), or hair in the stomach
(trichobezoar or hairball, more common in animals).

Mass of food in stomach   Gastric fundus

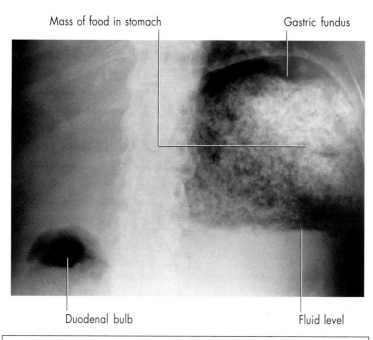

Duodenal bulb   Fluid level

Fig. 3.2 – Same patient: erect view.

Gastric neoplasms

Sometimes tumours may be visible in the fundus of the stomach on abdominal films and chest X-rays, this being an occasional presentation of gastric carcinoma.

Such an appearance must, however, be interpreted with great caution, as a physiologically contracted stomach can look very similar, the left lobe of a normal liver can indent the stomach here, and postoperatively fundoplication procedures produce filling defects medially that simulate abnormal masses. In the appropriate clinical setting (weight loss, anaemia, dyspepsia), however, patients causing concern over this appearance should be investigated.

Small bowel pathology usually manifests itself on plain X-rays by abnormal accumulations of gas and fluid, due to either functional (i.e. ileus) or truly mechanical obstruction. The main problem lies initially in trying to differentiate small bowel from large bowel.

Once the small bowel starts to dilate the small irregular pockets of gas that may be seen normally increase and coalesce, so that eventually the interior of the distended loops becomes completely outlined in continuity where the lumen is not occupied by fluid and complete mucosal folds appear.

Remember:

- The colon is peripheral and contains faeces and gas
- The small bowel is central and contains fluid and gas
- The more distal the obstruction, the more loops you will see
- The longer the duration of the obstruction, the bigger the fluid levels
- Fluid levels can only be seen on erect or decubitus films, and small fluid levels can occur normally
- It is not necessary to be obstructed to have fluid levels.

The standard series of films in the acute situation is a minimum of a supine abdomen and an erect chest X-ray. Experienced radiologists claim to make do with these alone, but most mortals are reassured by an erect abdomen as well.

NB The entire abdomen should be visualized, ideally on both the supine and erect films but certainly on the supine films from the top of the diaphragm to the hernial orifices in the groins, as these may be the site of an obstruction in an inguinal hernia. But remember that the presence of a hernia does not prove it is *causing* **an obstruction.** Two films may be required in each position to show the entire abdomen.

Look at (Fig. 3.3):

- The multiple centrally placed loops of bowel distended with gas
- The outlines of folds crossing the entire lumen in places
- The absence of any fluid levels.

Distended loops of small bowel   Stomach

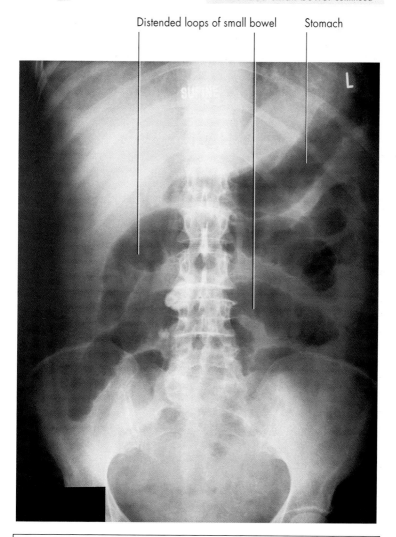

Fig. 3.3 – This is the supine abdominal radiograph of a patient presenting with abdominal pain, distension, nausea and vomiting. Note absence of fluid levels.

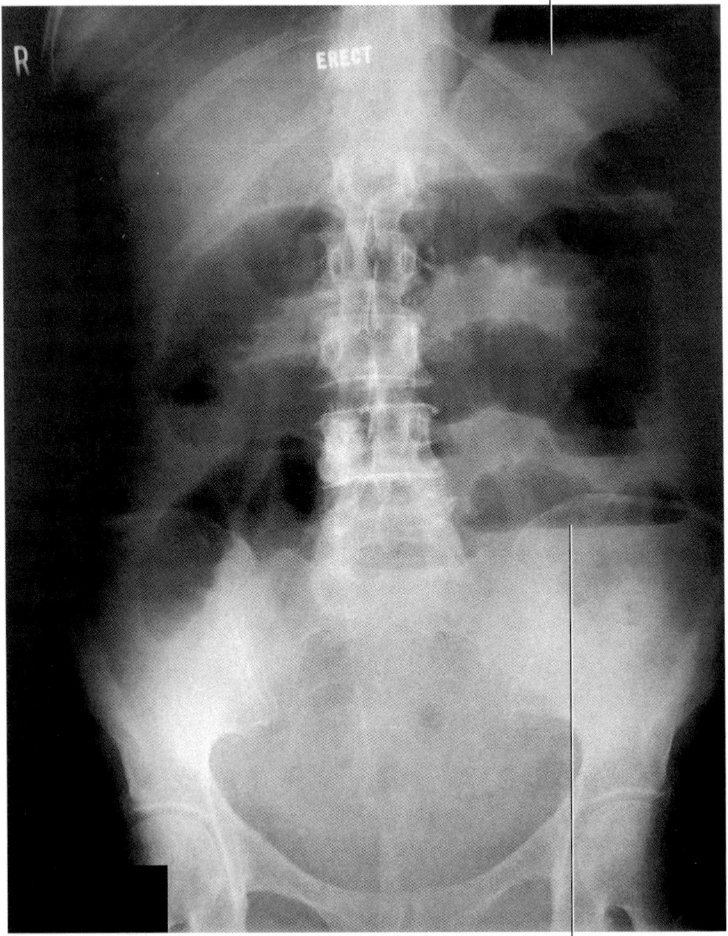

Gastric fluid level

R ERECT

Small bowel
fluid level

Fig. 3.4 – This is the same patient in the erect position. Note now the presence of fluid levels.

This (Fig. 3.4) is the classic appearance of a small bowel obstruction. The relatively small number of loops indicates a mid small bowel rather than a distal small bowel obstruction. The cause was adhesions from previous surgery some years before.

NB In order to demonstrate fluid levels you need fluid, overlying gas and a horizontal beam erect or decubitus film. Without the gas you won't see the fluid!

Although obstruction and perforation usually present separately and clinically differently, always check to make sure the patient has not sustained a perforation as a complication of an obstruction. This is a rare but important event.

NB The differential diagnosis of small bowel obstruction includes paralytic ileus and it may be hard to differentiate between the two on radiological grounds. The clinical context is usually crucially helpful, e.g. immediately postoperatively.

Remember: Both generalized and localized ileus may occur, e.g. the latter with 'sentinel loops' adjacent to an appendix abscess.

Causes of small bowel obstruction

- Postoperative adhesions (up to 80% of cases in western countries)
- Internal strangulation of bowel (band or internal hernia)
- External hernia (e.g. inguinal)
- Lymphoma
- Crohn's disease
- Intraluminal tumour
- Gallstone ileus (see page 64)
- Intussusception – usually children; in adults often associated with a tumour. Tends to begin in the ileum
- Congenital atresias – newborns.

Update: Recently spiral CT scanning of the abdomen has shown itself to be a very elegant way of demonstrating peritoneal adhesions causing obstruction, but the actual cause of most small bowel obstructions is not apparent from plain films alone.

Confounding factor: An inflamed or obstructed colon may contain fluid, in addition to the presence of small bowel fluid levels. Differentiating loops of small bowel from large bowel can then be exceptionally difficult.

Distended small bowel *continued*

A bit of epidemiology

As has already been stated, in the developed world, most small bowel intestinal obstruction is caused by adhesions. In places such as Africa, however, hernias are by far the most likely cause, as relatively little in the way of previous surgery will have been carried out to cause adhesions.

Vascular catastrophes

A mesenteric artery thrombosis or embolism is a critical event presenting as an acute abdomen. Radiologically the signs are those of ileus in the bowel, moving on to infarction and possibly gas formation in its walls. The clinical setting, e.g. atrial fibrillation, previous myocardial infarction etc., is important in suspecting this diagnosis. Occasionally mesenteric vein thrombosis will be the underlying cause associated with pancreatic carcinoma.

Ileus

Combined small and large bowel dilatation may form the classic radiological signs of paralytic ileus which, as stated, may be hard to differentiate from obstruction.

Causes

- Postoperative – after handling of the gut
- Hypokalaemia
- Drugs, e.g. L-dopa
- Intra-abdominal sepsis (peritonitis)
- Bowel infarction
- Trauma
- Reflex ileus from acute abdomen (renal colic, leaking aorta).

Gallstone ileus (a special form of obstruction)

This condition is recognized by abnormally distended gut and gas in an abnormal location, i.e. the biliary tract. It is in fact a misnomer, being due to genuine mechanical intestinal obstruction, caused by a large gallstone impacting in the gut, usually at the terminal ileum where the bowel is narrowest. This occurs usually after fistula formation between the gallbladder and the duodenum. It is one of the causes of intestinal obstruction where the actual cause may be inferred. Undiagnosed and untreated it carries a high mortality.

Look for (Fig. 3.5):

- Multiple dilated loops of small bowel, i.e. centrally placed loops where the folds go right across the lumen. The colon remains normal. This indicates small bowel obstruction.
- The number of distended loops: the more there are, the more distal the obstruction.
- Gas in the biliary tree. In this patient the entire bile duct is outlined and dilated. Gas is present in the lumen of the gallbladder. However, large recognizable quantities of gas will not always be present, and only in about a third of cases will the bile duct be fully displayed.
- The gallstone. Most commonly this is not seen, but may be located in the right iliac fossa or over the sacrum. It frequently consists of radiolucent cholesterol with only a thin calcified rim, making it hard to see, but in around 30% of patients it is visible. Most obstructing stones are over 1 inch (2.5 cm) in diameter, and may in fact be larger than they look if more cholesterol has been deposited beyond the calcified rim. If the patient was previously known to have had a gallstone in the gallbladder, look to see if it has gone from that location.

NB No stone was visible in this patient.

Causes of gas in the biliary tree

- Previous biliary surgery, e.g. Whipple's operation or anastomoses to the gut
- Instrumentation, e.g. ERCP/sphincterotomy
- Fistula formation, e.g. gallstone ileus
- Posterior perforation of an ulcer
- Malignant spread to the bile duct
- Emphysematous cholecystitis (diabetics)
- Lax sphincter (physiological).

Gas outlining gall bladder   Gas in bile duct   Solid faeces in colon   Dilated small bowel

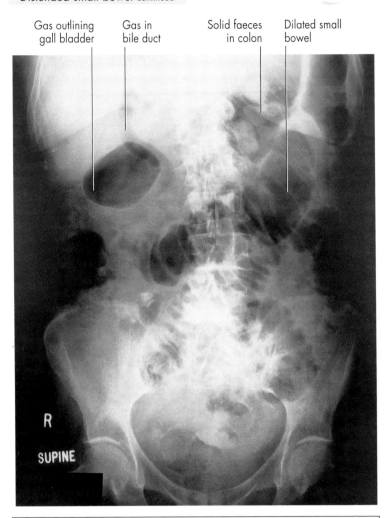

R

SUPINE

*Fig. 3.5 – **Gallstone ileus** This is a supine AP abdominal X-ray of a 55-year-old woman with a history of right upper quadrant pain, who now presents with more severe pain, fever, nausea and vomiting. The X-ray shows distended small bowel and gas in the bile ducts. You can also see gas in the gallbladder.*

Figures 3.6 and 3.7 show a distal large bowel obstruction caused by a carcinoma of the descending colon in an elderly woman who presented late with rectal bleeding, weight loss and, latterly, increasing swelling of the abdomen.

Colonic obstruction can assume a number of appearances, depending on the position of the obstruction and whether or not the ileocaecal valve is competent. If it is, the caecum, being the most distensible part of the large bowel, will distend, but if not the back-pressure will be transmitted through the valve into the small bowel, and that too will distend, as in a small bowel obstruction, but without caecal distension.

Distension of both of these parts of the bowel together can of course occur without obstruction, owing to ileus, and isolated colonic distension ('colonic pseudo-obstruction') may also occur associated with medical conditions such as MI (myocardial infarction), and the radiologist may be asked to exclude organic obstruction by running in some contrast medium retrogradely. The critical diameter for the caecum is 9 cm, beyond which it is in great danger of perforation.

Look for:

- Dilated loops (>6 cm)
- Marked distension of the caecum
- General peripheral position of bowel
- Several incomplete haustral folds, typical of the colon, and a few complete ones — normal variation!
- Fluid faeces on the left (erect film), indicating colonic malfunction
- Involvement down to the level of the descending colon
- A lack of distension of the small bowel, indicating a competent ileocaecal valve.

NB Most colonic obstructions in the UK are caused by tumours (up to 60%), but in some other countries torsion of the bowel (volvulus) is the commonest cause.

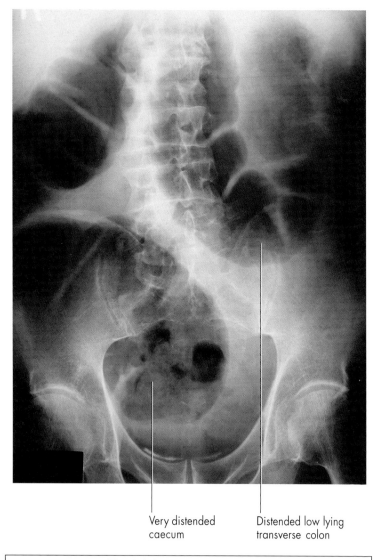

Very distended
caecum

Distended low lying
transverse colon

Fig. 3.6 – Supine AP film of abdomen. Female patient aged 72, presenting with severe abdominal distension. Note the absence of fluid levels.

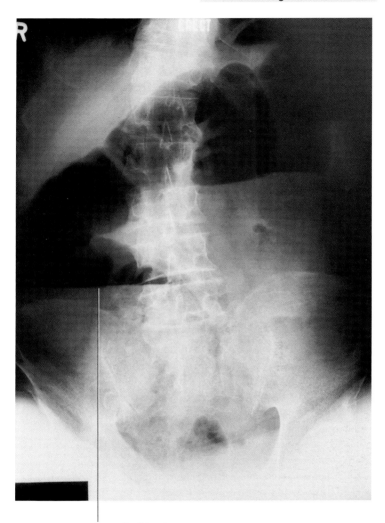

Large fluid level in
ascending colon

Fig. 3.7 – Same patient showing big fluid levels in the erect position.

Causes of large bowel obstruction

- Carcinomas (unlike the small bowel, where adhesions are the most common cause)
- Diverticular disease
- Volvulus – most commonly sigmoid and caecum (see below) in parts of the bowel with a long mesentery
- Inflammatory bowel disease (e.g. Crohn's)
- Appendix abscess
- Metastases
- Lymphoma
- Pelvic masses.

Causes of colonic pseudo-obstruction (may require contrast study to exclude true obstruction and intervention to decompress caecum)

- MI (with pulmonary oedema)
- Pneumonia
- Myxoedema.

Abdominal hernias

Apart from being an interesting incidental finding, the presence of external hernias is important because they may be the site of intestinal obstruction. From the diagnostic radiological point of view the most significant application of this knowledge lies in ensuring that when a patient presents with intestinal obstruction the inguinal and femoral regions are clearly demonstrated on the films – preferably in both the erect and the supine positions.

If an obese patient has a strangulated hernia in the region of the groin this may be a good way to help confirm it.

NB The presence of a hernia in the context of intestinal obstruction does not prove that the hernia is the cause of the obstruction. However, if there is directional continuity of a loop of bowel straight towards a cut-off segment of gut in a hernia, for example, true cause and effect are most likely. Remember, if a herniated loop of bowel does not contain gas it will not be visible.

Scrotal hernias

Appearance of hernias in the groin

Look for:

- Loops of gas-filled bowel extending below the level of the inguinal ligaments on both sides
- Continuity of these loops with another loop in the true pelvis
- Enlargement of the scrotum to accommodate these loops (auscultation of the scrotum may render bowel sounds audible).

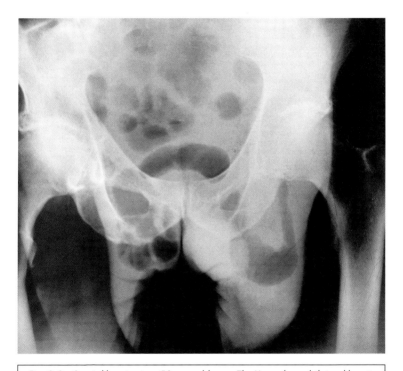

Fig. 3.8 – Scrotal hernias in a 50-year-old man. The X-ray shows bilateral hernia formation in the groin, extending into the scrotum. This was an incidental finding and the patient was not obstructed at the time.

Look at (Fig. 3.9):

- The massive scrotum containing multiple gas/liquid levels
- Longitudinal fluid levels, indicating that this is a decubitus film (patient lying on his right side).

Causes of massive scrotal enlargement are rare. Filariasis is one, but herniation of bowel is another. It is this sort of gross pathology that gives rise to the old medical jokes about patients having to carry their scrotums around in a wheelbarrow!

Do not forget:

- A Richter's hernia may be causing a severe obstruction at the inguinal level with only a small partial knuckle of bowel inside it.
- Hernias can occur in other locations, e.g. at and around the umbilicus, and contain small and/or large bowel.
- Internal hernias can also occur – for instance into the lesser sac.

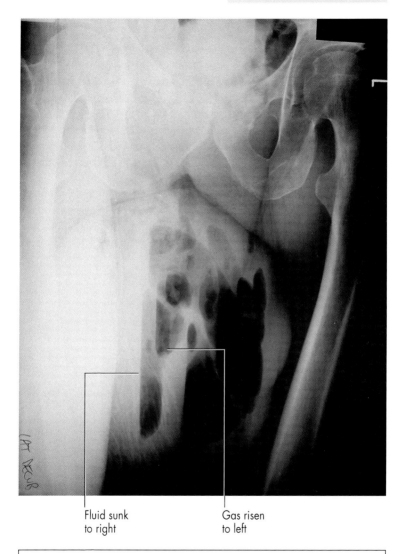

Fluid sunk   Gas risen
to right   to left

Fig. 3.9 – A patient with a huge scrotal hernia. NB This is a decubitus film with the patient lying on his right side and large fluid levels present with the gas lying uppermost.

Look for (Fig. 3.10):

- The characteristic appearance of inspissated faecal matter – rounded masses of mottled or granular texture – due to tiny pockets of gas which they always contain. Find these and you've found the colon.
- Larger quantities of surrounding gas, with occasional haustral folds crossing part of the lumen and outward-billowing folds primarily in the periphery of the abdomen. The transverse colon may, however, be very tortuous and dip down towards the pelvis as it does here.
- Formed faeces in the right side of the colon. This usually indicates constipation, as the material here is usually fluid, mobile and amorphous.
- Distension and loading of the rectum and sigmoid (not in this patient). But these too can be grossly distended in severe constipation. In some individuals the colon may be distended to truly enormous proportions e.g. institutionalized patients who are relatively asymptomatic but who pose considerable anxiety when first X-rayed.

Causes of constipation

- Painful conditions – anal fissure, haemorrhoids
- Social – irregular work patterns, hospitalization, travel (long flights)
- Psychological – institutionalized individuals/defectives, depression
- Elderly – immobility, poor diet, altered routines
- Colonic disease – carcinoma, slow transit, excessively long colon
- Postoperative – childbirth, pelvic floor repair
- Paraplegia – autonomic dysfunction
- Drugs – analgesics, opiates, antidepressants, iron
- Parkinsonism – retardation
- Hypothyroid disease – generalized reduction in bodily functions
- Chagas' disease – trypanosomiasis infection with megacolon
- Hirschsprung's disease, in children. In this condition look for huge mottled masses and gas in the surrounding periphery of the colon.

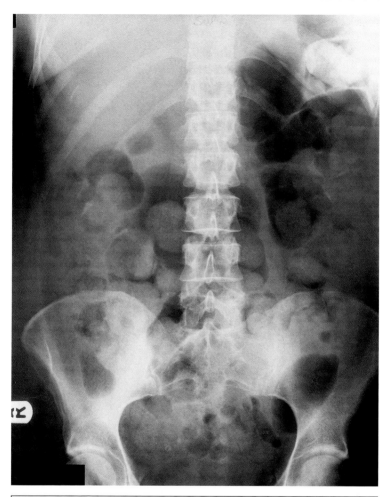

Fig. 3.10 – **Constipation** This is a 55-year-old woman who presented with increasing abdominal pain, distension, and complaints of reduced bowel frequency. You can see faecal overloading in the large bowel.

Appendicitis is the most common acute surgical emergency, but most appendices are not visible on abdominal X-rays.

Often the diagnosis and treatment are straightforward, but occasionally difficult or atypical presentations occur and under these circumstances abdominal films may be helpful. First check that any woman of reproductive age is not pregnant, as appendicitis often occurs in the young, i.e. ask about the LMP: your patient may have dysmenorrhoea.

NB A normal X-ray does not exclude appendicitis and no one radiological sign confirms it. However, when certain radiological signs occur together in the appropriate clinical setting, the likelihood of appendicitis being the correct diagnosis greatly increases.

A word about pathology

Appendicitis is caused by blockage of the mouth of this organ with inspissated faeces or a calcified mass thereof (faecolith), leading to distension and infection, surrounding inflammatory reaction, bowel stasis and potential rupture – reflected over time from normality to established radiological changes.

This (Fig. 3.11) is appendicitis complicated by abscess formation.

Look for:

- Calcified faecoliths. These may occur in normal people but also occur in around 14% of patients with acute appendicitis, and as they grow may take on a laminated appearance. They are different from calcified lymph nodes. A cluster of four faecoliths is present here.

- Mass effect around the appendix. The bowel loops are displaced away from the primary focus of infection due to oedema, rupture and abscess formation, with walling off by the greater omentum – 'the abdominal policeman'.

- Distended loops of bowel – 'sentinel loops'. These are due to localized ileus from the inflammation or matting with adhesions, going on to complete intestinal obstruction. It is the adjacent colon that is distended here.

Faecolith

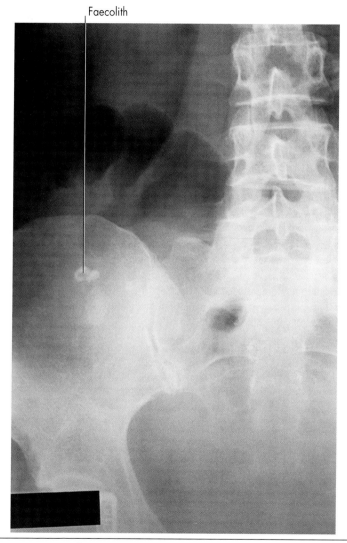

Fig. 3.11 – Localised view of erect film of a patient with abdominal pain commencing centrally and then localizing to the right iliac fossa, followed by increasing toxicity, fever and a palpable mass in the lower right abdomen and tenderness PR on the right.

Another appendicitis

This (Fig. 3.12) is the lower right quadrant detail from the film of a 60-year-old febrile patient with initial central abdominal pain, later localizing to the lower right.

Look at:

- The curved C-shaped object in the right flank
- The black density of its interior.

This is gas in the lumen of an inflamed and turgid appendix. It is a rare sign and must be interpreted with caution, as it may also occur in normal people.

Other radiological signs to look for in appendicitis include:

- Free gas – a very serious sign of perforation – either intraperitoneally or in the retroperitoneum (the appendix can lie in either space), but this is rare.
- Loss of the right psoas margin, but again this is a non-specific sign.
- Flexion or scoliosis concave to the affected side. This is nature's way of relieving spasm in the muscles on the painful side. It may also be seen in trauma or renal colic, but does not always occur.
- Other indirect signs of inflammation/intra-abdominal pathology causing loss of clarity to the right properitoneal fat stripe in the flank. Much is often made of this sign.

But:

- This area should be included on abdominal films but often it is not.
- You will often need a bright light to see it, but often it is too dark to see anyway even when the relevant area is included.

Other radiological manifestations of the appendix

- Remember that the appendix may retain barium from a recent enema or oral barium study for many weeks or months. Failure to fill does not necessarily indicate disease; also, most patients are nil-by-mouth as emergencies, thereby precluding oral barium as a test, although were it to fill up with contrast that would rule out appendicitis as the cause, thus requiring alternative pathology to be sought.

Point of interest: Colonic diverticula may retain barium for many weeks or months after a barium enema or meal, causing possibly dozens of very dense

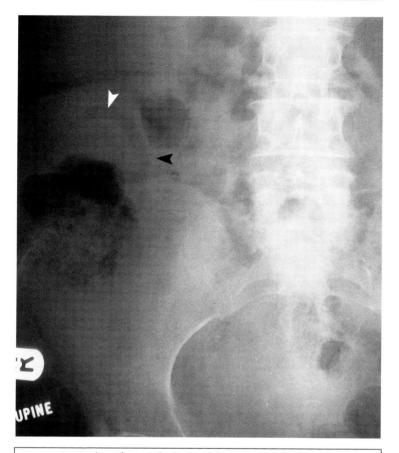

Fig. 3.12 – Finding of gas in the lumen of the appendix (arrows).

opacities around the colon. If you can see what looks like this, look in the notes or X-ray packet for the culprit.

Remember: Retained barium from radiological studies is a rare but recognized cause of appendicitis.

Footnote: Non-invasive preoperative imaging assessment for appendicitis may now be sought by ultrasound and CT, looking for an appendicolith, a distended appendix >6mm in diameter, and surrounding inflammatory signs of oedema or fluid.

Volvulus or 'twisting' can affect any part of the intra-abdominal gastrointestinal tract, including the stomach and small bowel, but this is relatively rare.

More common, but still relatively rare compared with all other causes of obstruction of the large bowel, is volvulus of the sigmoid colon and the caecum in western countries, although it tends to be more frequent in Africa, for example.

Sigmoid volvulus

This (Fig. 3.13) usually occurs in elderly patients who have redundant loops of sigmoid colon on a long mesentery and a history of constipation. Subacute manifestations or vague symptoms may occur but in the acute form the patient may become severely ill with abdominal pain, complete constipation and, on PR, an empty rectum. Delay in diagnosis may lead to ischaemia, gangrene, perforation and death.

Look for:

- A grossly distended loop of sigmoid colon extending from the pelvis to under the diaphragm. Compression together of the two medial walls produces the 'coffee bean sign'. Erect films may show excessive quantities of gas relative to fluid > 2:1.
- A lack of haustra. These are effaced by the enormous distension, but other loops of colon underlying it may simulate haustra in the distended loop.
- Apex above the 10th vertebra in the thoracic spine, again a measure of the severity of distension that occurs in a true volvulus. This point is off the top of this film, which was only one of several needed to demonstrate the entire abdomen and chest.
- Convergence of lower margins of the distended loops on the left.
- Liver overlap sign – indicative of the degree of distension of the bowel, i.e. a colonic loop to the height of the liver or above it on the right.
- Left flank overlap sign – indicative of distension of the same, i.e. the left limb of the 'coffee bean' overlies the descending colon, which may be seen behind it.
- 'Free air' – sign of perforation (not present here yet).

These are the classic signs of a sigmoid volvulus, but in some patients the radiological signs are atypical and therefore less obvious. Retrograde running-in of contrast medium per rectum may show a twisted beak-like or 'bird of prey' sign at the point of convergence of the distended loops and confirm the diagnosis.

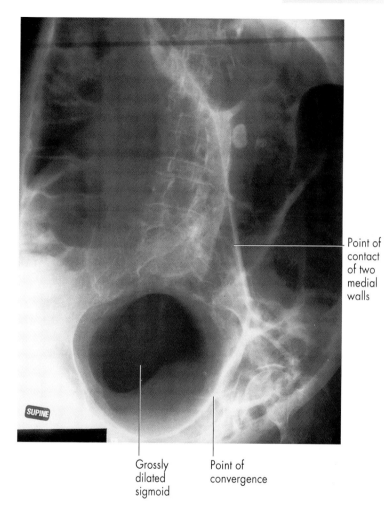

Point of contact of two medial walls

Grossly dilated sigmoid

Point of convergence

Fig. 3.13 – Supine AP radiograph. Sigmoid volvulus. An elderly institutionalized woman aged 76 with an acute exacerbation of long-standing intermittent abdominal symptoms of pain and distension, and prior constipation. Note the distended sigmoid. This is the famous 'coffee bean' sign.

This condition may respond initially to endoscopic tubal manipulation and decompression, but most will recur. Definitive surgery with partial colonic resection may then be required.

Perforation and gangrene constitute an acute emergency and require immediate surgical intervention.

Inflammatory bowel disease

It is not the job of plain film radiology to establish the diagnosis of mild inflammatory bowel disease, which requires tissue biopsy, but rather to evaluate patients presenting with exacerbations or complications thereof, and other than in obstruction it plays little part in the assessment of small bowel disease, for which barium studies are required. The normal colon, however, usually contains semifluid faecal matter on the right-hand side and more solid faecal matter on the left-hand side.

In suspected inflammatory large bowel disease therefore look for:

An absence of formed faecal matter in the left-hand side of the colon.

This indicates that the colon is not carrying out its function properly, i.e. storing its contents for a sufficiently long time and absorbing water from them, and these patients will usually have a history of diarrhoea.

Diarrhoea of course has many causes (see opposite), including gastrointestinal tract infections and the use of aperients e.g. in the preparation of patients for radiological procedures. At times this can be so marked as to produce a virtually faeces-free and 'gasless' abdomen.

The patient's history – e.g. of recent foreign travel, self-medication or the medical use of suppositories etc. – therefore becomes paramount.

Causes of diarrhoea

These are conveniently divided into acute and chronic.

Acute

- Infections, e.g. gastroenteritis, food poisoning
- Dietary excesses: lager and hot curries!
- Traveller's diarrhoea due to *E.coli, Entamoeba, Shigella* etc.

Note: The 'gasless' abdomen, where the X-ray shows a lack of faecal matter and almost total absence of gas, may indicate early obstruction, diarrhoea or laxative use.

Chronic

- Inflammatory bowel disease (Crohn's, ulcerative colitis)
- Malabsorption
- Infection (parasites)
- Malignancy in bowel
- GI surgery (vagotomy, partial bowel resection, blind loops etc.)
- Constipation (in the elderly) with 'overflow diarrhoea' and rectal plug
- Laxatives
- Endocrine causes
    pancreatic insufficiency
    pancreatic neoplasm
    thyrotoxicosis
    diabetic autonomic neuropathy.

Complications of inflammatory bowel disease

Small bowel

This usually involves Crohn's disease and plain films may show intestinal obstruction or signs of fistula formation leading, for example, to air in the urinary tract (bladder, ureter, renal pelvis) or the biliary system (i.e. bile duct). Rarely malignancy may supervene.

Large bowel

Look for (Fig. 3.14):

- The generalized lack of formed faecal matter
- The oedematous folds of mucosa, especially in the transverse colon.

This is called 'thumbprinting' and is usually a manifestation of acute and severe inflammation in the colon due to ulcerative colitis. There are, however, many causes of thumbprinting, the more common ones including:

- Crohn's disease
- Ischaemic colitis
- Intramural haematoma
- Metastases
- Lymphoma
- Pseudomembranous colitis
- Allergic reactions ('colonic hives').

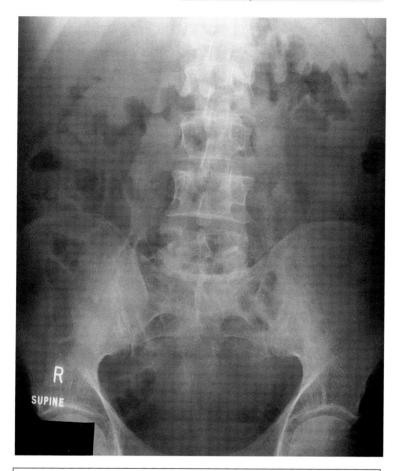

Fig. 3.14 – A 43-year-old man with acute diarrhoea passing slime and bleeding per rectum. This is a supine AP film showing an acute exacerbation of ulcerative colitis.

This (Fig. 3.15) is a case of toxic megacolon or toxic dilatation of the colon. Look for:

- Generalized or localized dilatation of the lumen of the bowel (> 6 cm)
- Lobulated masses in the lumen (inflammatory pseudopolyps)
- Excessive gas
- Absent faeces (note that the intraluminal masses are smooth and contain no mottling due to pockets of gas)
- Gas in the wall of the bowel (not present here, but may indicate imminent perforation)
- Evidence of free gas – pneumoperitoneum – 'double wall sign' if the bowel has perforated. Not present here
- Evidence of gas in the portal vein. Not present here. When present this is usually an antemortem event.

Toxic dilatation of the colon is an acute surgical emergency and this patient required an emergency colectomy, which was carried out forthwith.

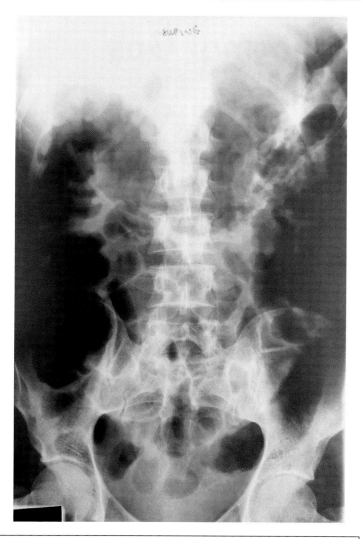

Fig. 3.15 – This is a 35-year-old man who was admitted in a state of shock with bloody diarrhoea. He had a history of ulcerative colitis.

Chapter 4

Abnormal Gas

- Gas is the body's own natural contrast medium and its appearance as the darkest density appearing on X-ray films should now be familiar to you, especially in the abdomen as well as in the chest.

- Most of the time it is confined to the lumen of the gut, where you can make great use of it to deduce the diameter, and mucosal state of the bowel wall. However, the problem is:

  (a) that the gut is usually undergoing peristalsis of varying degrees, so that

  (b) enormously variable quantities of gas may be present from patient to patient and from time to time, both of which tax the observer to try and interpret correctly. Often only *parts* of the bowel are visible.

  (c) adherent faecal residue may simulate mucosal abnormality in the colon, as may residual food in the stomach.

- Much less frequently, but most importantly from the diagnostic viewpoint, owing to a variety of pathological processes gas may escape from the lumen of the gut into the peritoneal cavity, as well as into the retroperitoneal space.

- More subtly, it may track into the wall of the bowel itself and, by fistula formation, further break into other systems such as the urinary or biliary tracts, or even out onto the surface of the skin (enterocutaneous fistula). Gas may also track down into the abdomen from the chest, form in abscesses as a result of infection with gas-producing organisms, appear in vessels such as the portal vein as a preterminal event, and also appear as a result of iatrogenic activities such as embolization procedures (e.g. in the kidney).

- It must be understood that extraluminal intraperitoneal gas is to be expected after surgery, laparoscopy or peritoneal dialysis, so that the radiologist *must* be given the relevant clinical information and not be misled into diagnosing pathology incorrectly as a result of failure by the clinician to provide it.

- Conversely, after an iatrogenic procedure such as endoscopy extraluminal gas should not be expected, and its presence in that situation indicates a catastrophe, i.e. perforation of the gut. **The procedure need not have been technically difficult for this to occur.**

Pneumoperitoneum

The radiological signs of a pneumoperitoneum are among the most important signs in radiology, indeed in medicine. Sometimes the amount of free gas is small and you may have to work to demonstrate it. **Miss it and the patient may die.**
  Look for:

- Bilateral dark crescents of gas under both hemidiaphragms. NB Figure 4.1 was taken erect, so the gas has risen. This is a large pneumoperitoneum, but small amounts of gas require time to rise to the subdiaphragmatic position so it is a good idea to leave the patient upright for 10 minutes to allow this to happen before taking the X-ray
- Gas may appear on one side of the abdomen only, usually the right
- No gas may be seen if the perforation has been sealed off by the omentum
- If only a small amount of gas is present it may be missed unless the film is centred at the level of the diaphragms – usually a chest is centred around the fourth thoracic vertebra. With attention to detail as little as 1ml of free gas may be demonstrated.

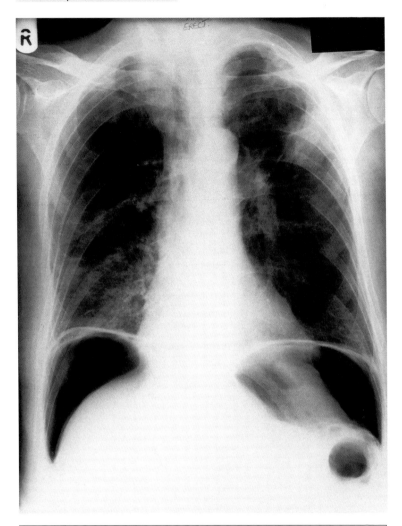

Fig. 4.1 – B.L. Erect chest film. 60-year-old patient with a history of ulcer disease, presenting with acute abdominal pain and board-like rigidity in the abdomen. Note the bilateral radiolucent collections of gas under each hemidiaphragm. This was due to a perforated duodenal ulcer. There is also a mass in the left lung.

Supine films will usually have been taken routinely with the erect ones, and certain more subtle signs of free gas in the peritoneal cavity have been described to enable the diagnosis to be established under these circumstances.

Look for:

- 'The double-wall' sign (Fig. 4.2), i.e. both sides of the wall of loops of bowel become visible because of air on the inside and air on the outside – try to find an isolated viscus such as the stomach or bowel loop, but remember that closely apposed loops may give a false positive 'double-wall' sign
- 'Football or dome sign'. With a large pneumoperitoneum the undersurface of the diaphragm may be surrounded by air, giving a dark dome-like appearance in the upper abdomen even on supine films
- Visualization of falciform ligament – 'Silver's sign'
- Gas in the scrotum in children
- In seriously ill patients the use of erect films may not be possible and decubitus films with the left side down centred on the right upper flank should be taken.

Bright lights may be required to see this area properly, as for technical reasons the films often come out very dark in this situation.

Gas at falciform ligament

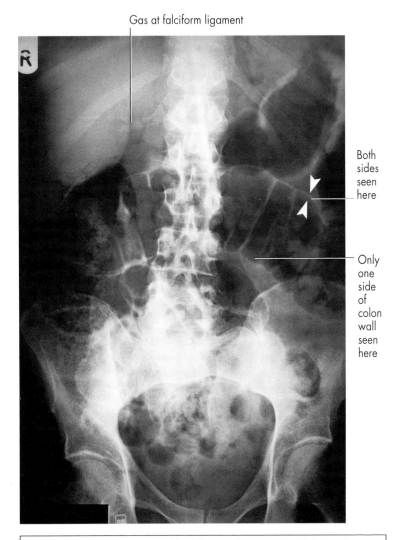

Both sides seen here

Only one side of colon wall seen here

4.2 – Pneumoperitoneum – 'double-wall' sign. This is a supine abdomen showing some of the more subtle signs of a pneumoperitoneum.

The causes of a pneumoperitoneum are legion and are often divided into those with clinical signs of peritonitis and those without, although some of the latter may later develop signs of peritonitis.

Crucial fact: Special vigilance must be exercised in dealing with patients on larger doses of steroids. These drugs both predispose the patient to erosion and perforation of the upper GI tract and then mask the symptoms and signs. The diagnosis of perforation then relies entirely on the X-ray, so a high index of suspicion for this phenomenon must be maintained.

Note (Fig. 4.2):

- The diaphragms are not visible, nor any gas beneath them
- Free gas, however, is definitely present as both the inside and outside walls of parts of the colon are visible, i.e. the 'double-wall' sign
- Gas is tracking up the falciform ligament.

Causes of a pneumoperitoneum

With peritonitis

- Perforated peptic ulcer (stomach or duodenum)
- Intestinal obstruction
- Ruptured diverticular disease
- Penetrating injury – gunshots, knife-wounds etc.
- Ruptured inflammatory bowel disease (e.g. megacolon)
- Colonic infections (typhoid).

Without peritonitis

- Post laparotomy
- Post laparoscopy
- Jejunal diverticulosis
- Steroids
- Tracking from chest (pneumothorax)
- Peritoneal dialysis
- Vaginal insufflation (douching, squatting, oral sex, postpartum exercises, water-skiing)
- Pneumatosis coli.

Many important phenomena can simulate a pneumoperitoneum and lead to misdiagnosis and unnecessary surgery, with all its medical and medico-legal complications. A good selection of these is shown to emphasize their crucial importance.

Linear atelectasis (Fig. 4.3)

- Linear atelectasis is a phenomenon that occurs in the lungs, usually at the bases.

- It is frequently associated with infection or pulmonary embolism and is commonly seen after anaesthetics in the postoperative state. It forms dense horizontal or curved bands which may simulate the diaphragm.

- Note how the band at the right costophrenic angle curves up instead of down. Normally it resolves within days or weeks, but may persist for longer.

Note (Fig. 4.4, p. 94):

- The band of increased density running just above the medial part of the right hemidiaphragm, creating a lucent view of the air in the lung beneath it and simulating a pneumoperitoneum.

- This is a more subtle example of linear atelectasis following anaesthesia. Nothing had been done to the abdomen.

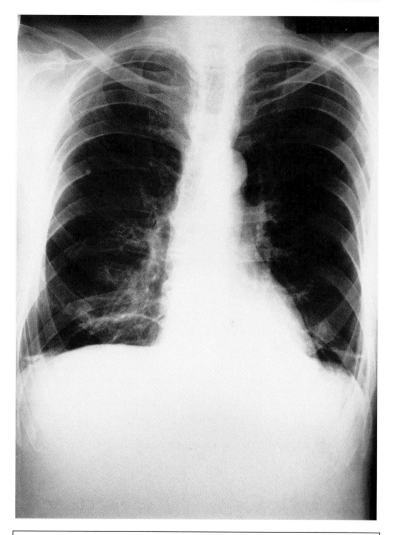

Fig. 4.3 – This is a case of bilateral linear atelectasis simulating a pneumoperitoneum.

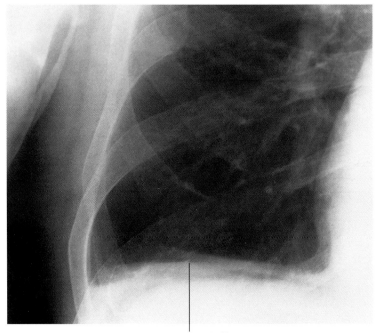

Band of linear atelectasis

Fig. 4.4 – This is a postoperative general anaesthetic patient who has just had ENT surgery. Detail from right base of a chest X-ray.

Chilaiditi's syndrome – colonic interposition

Note (Fig. 4.5):

- The incidental finding of pockets of gas beneath the right hemidiaphragm
- Multiple bands of mucosal folds indicating gut. This is colonic interposition. An abdominal film showed continuity with the rest of the colon
- Rarely the small bowel may interpose as well
- This may be intermittent in nature, i.e. present on one occasion and gone the next.

It may be seen with shrunken livers (cirrhosis), in COPD with a large thoracic

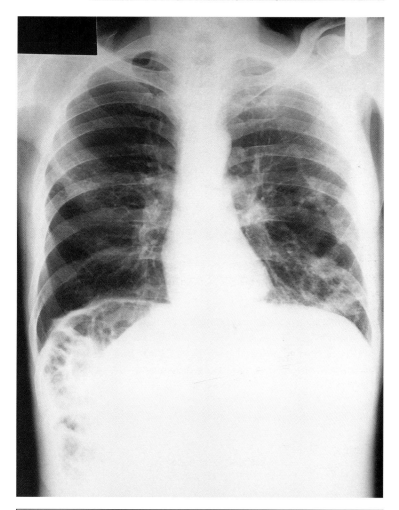

Fig. 4.5 –**Chilaiditi's syndrome** Colonic interposition. This is the chest X-ray of a 60-year-old male with chronic lung disease.

outlet, postoperatively when the surgeon has pushed the gut out of the way to get at something else, or spontaneously.

Meteorism

Look for (Fig. 4.6):

- Excessive air swallowing often associated with crying, especially in children, causing gut distended with gas to crowd up underneath both hemi-diaphragms. (Interposition again on the right.)
- Folds of the bowel crossing the gas-filled lumen, confirming the presence of gut
- Superimposition of bowel loops
- Continuity of loops with others in the abdomen.

This is meteorism. There were no abdominal symptoms and no perforation.

Subphrenic abscess (see Fig. 4.15)

Look for:

- Fluid levels under either hemidiaphragm, more commonly the right.

This usually occurs postoperatively in a very sick patient. Part of the gas will often have been generated by organisms and will not all be residual from the laparotomy. Ultrasound may be very helpful in demonstrating fluid, but will tend to be blocked by any gas that is present. CT may then be required. Plain X-rays, however, often first alert one to the diagnosis.

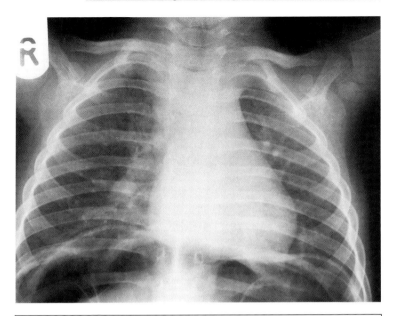

Fig. 4.6 – **Child with meteorism** *This is the X-ray of a young child with a suspected chest infection who had been crying profusely before the film was taken.*

- Skin folds, especially in the elderly, infants and severely dehydrated patients
- Cortical rib margins overlapping diaphragms
- Lobulated diaphragm with gut underneath one or more humps.

This is a matter for careful inspection and analysis of the films.

NB When there is doubt about a pneumoperitoneum or demonstrating the site of a leak is required, oral water-soluble contrast (but not barium) can be given to try and demonstrate a perforation, under screening control by a radiologist. Barium should not be used as it is harmful and dangerous should it escape through a perforation into the peritoneal cavity, exacerbating infection and causing barium granulomata.

NB Just occasionally one or other of these phenomena can coexist with a genuine pneumoperitoneum. Dual pathology is by no means unheard of.

Fat beneath the diaphragm

Look for (Fig. 4.7):

- Constant radiolucent stripe beneath the left hemidiaphragm
- Constancy in the size, shape and position over time and no movement with change of position, e.g. a decubitus film
- Associated cardiophrenic fat pad at the apex of the heart.

This is a lipoperitoneum, i.e. a collection of fat beneath the left hemidiaphragm. Note its similarity to a genuine pneumoperitoneum. A lipoperitoneum is more likely to occur in an obese patient or one with a cardiophrenic fat pad indicating tendency to form excess body fat. The lucent line however is not quite so dark as gas giving an important clue to the diagnosis.

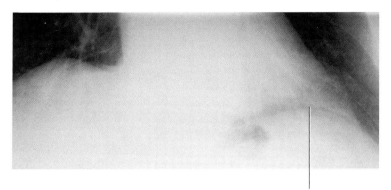

Lucent stripe of fat simulating a pneumoperitoneum

Fig. 4.7 – Detail from one of a number of identical chest X-rays taken on this patient over several years.

Distended gastric fundus

This can form an extensive quantity of air apparently beneath the left hemidiaphragm.

Look for:

- A fluid level in the erect position, as seen on most normal chest X-rays
- Typical disposition of the stomach in continuity with gastric fundus on supine film
- The total thickness of the left hemidiaphragm. A 'naked' diaphragm with free air on either side of it measures only 2–3 mm. With the thickness of the gastric fundal wall beneath it the total thickness will approximate to more like 4–5 mm in total. Proceed with caution, however, as exceptions can occur.

On occasion gas may collect in the retroperitoneal space and cause a so-called **pneumoretroperitoneum.** However, it is usually due to rupture of parts of the gut with retroperitoneal components, e.g. the duodenum or rectum, either spontaneously due to pathology or following instrumentation, such as endoscopy, or penetrating injury (e.g. a stab wound).

At one time the deliberate introduction of gas into the retroperitoneum was carried out as a diagnostic procedure, by inserting a needle through the perineum and injecting carbon dioxide – 'presacral pneumography' – to demonstrate renal or adrenal masses, but this is now completely obsolete. Nevertheless this illustration of the technique shows well what to expect and what you will see when it occurs.

Note:

- The intense black density surrounding the psoas muscle margins, the kidneys, adrenals and spleen
- Marked enlargement of the right adrenal and spleen
- Associated gas in the peritoneal cavity, which may or may not (as here) be present.

NB Gas in the retroperitoneum is a serious radiological sign and requires urgent assessment to find its cause, although the preceding history is usually obvious.

NB A lack of gas under either hemidiaphragm on erect films does not exclude a perforation, and air in the retroperitoneum will not necessarily be associated with air under either hemidiaphragm. A posteriorly perforating ulcer may lead to air only in the retroperitoneum. In *massive* perforations free gas may readily be seen under both hemidiaphragms, even on *supine* films.

Often, however, retroperitoneal gas is present only in small quantities and constitutes a subtle radiological finding.

But do not mistake streaks of dirt in the erector spinal muscles for retroperitoneal gas in the elderly.

Right
adrenal

Very dark
retroperitoneal
gas

Spleen

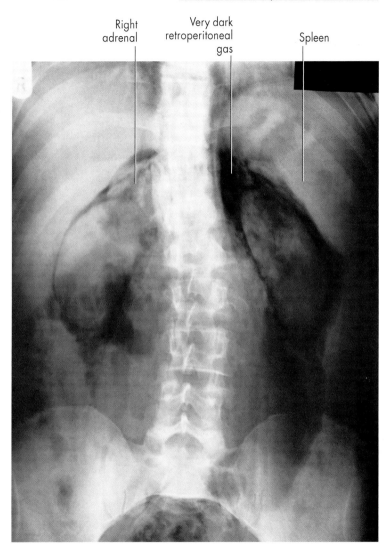

Fig. 4.8 – Retroperitoneal gas – old X-ray from a deliberate case of 'presacral pnuemography'. Note the intense 'negative contrast' highlighting of the kidneys. Note also the enlarged spleen and big right adrenal gland.

There are some important facts worth emphasizing about these films. Free gas in the abdomen is normal after surgery and usually diminishes day by day on the early supine films. If the amount of gas does not diminish it may indicate the breakdown of an anastomosis or leakage from the site of recent surgery.

After several days, when the patient is feeling better and sat up, the gas rises, and it may then appear that a lot more of it is suddenly present underneath the diaphragms when previous supine or semirecumbent films are compared with erect ones. Remember this phenomenon and monitor it before misdiagnosing a 'leak'. The patient's clinical state will be a good guide.

Tips:

- Take advantage of any view of the lung bases you get on abdominal films. The amount of energy required to demonstrate the abdomen is much greater than for a chest X-ray, and lung bases that 'cannot be shown' due to obesity or poor inspiration on conventional chest X-rays may show up particularly well on abdominal films – for basal atelectasis, effusions, cavities, metastases etc.

- Asking for 'an upper abdominal film' may be a subtle way of getting the radiographer to show the lung bases for you.

- On postoperative films look particularly closely for signs of left lower lobe and linear collapse. Colonic interposition may also occur postoperatively.

- Do not forget to look extremely critically at the position of all tubes, drains, stents and coils that may have been put into the abdomen and maintain a high index of suspicion for signs of infection, ileus, etc.

- Remember early post-operative films may have to be done on mobile machines and be technically less satisfactory and more prone to artefacts.

This has already been touched on under gallstone ileus. Remember, the gallbladder and bile duct are not routinely visible on plain X-rays and, when illustrated in texts, have usually been injected with contrast medium so that they show up white. It is important, however, to learn to identify familiar anatomical structures presenting in an unfamiliar way, that is, when outlined by gas. This is known as 'negative contrast'.

The clinical state of the patient will be a good guide as to the potential seriousness of finding gas on X-ray in the biliary tree, e.g. very sick with gas-forming organism infection, or clinically well due to previous choledocho-duodenostomy surgery.

In the past carbonated drinks have been given to children with bile ducts anastomosed to the gut to fill them with CO_2 and monitor their subsequent size – a form of 'coca-colagram'– thereby avoiding the risks of iodinated contrast. Ultrasound would now be used, however, and can detect gas by bright echoes coming from the bile ducts.

Gas in the wall of the gallbladder

As opposed to gas in its lumen, gas can occur in the wall of the gallbladder itself– so-called 'emphysematous cholecystitis'– due to infection with gas-forming organisms, especially in diabetics. It looks similar to gas in the wall of the urinary bladder (see Fig. 4.12). Other than those stated on page 63, causes of gas in the biliary tree include:

- Crohn's disease
- Pancreatitis
- Parasites, e.g. ascariasis.

As with gas in the biliary tract, the finding of gas in the urinary tract usually indicates recent instrumentation or else something serious going on, such as gas-forming infection or fistula formation.

Causes of gas in bladder lumen (see X-ray on p. 182)

- Iatrogenic, e.g. cystoscopy
- Due to fistula formation.

Causes of bladder fistula

- Malignancy of bowel, bladder, genital system
- Crohn's disease
- Diverticular disease
- Postoperatively ('controlled trauma')
- Trauma (uncontrolled)
- Radiotherapy
- Foreign body
- Ulcerative colitis.

Note (Fig. 4.9):

- The distension of both collecting systems from the obstructing effect of the bladder carcinoma
- The white outline of the left renal collecting system by contrast medium – the usual 'positive contrast' from the i.v. injection
- The black outline of the right renal collecting system, i.e. 'negative contrast' from intrapelvic and intracalcyeal gas on this side, plus the non-function of the right kidney.

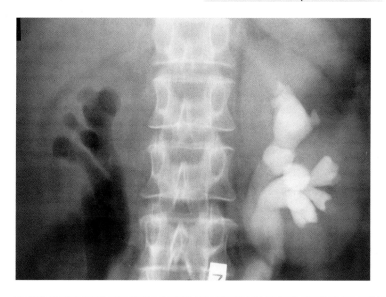

Fig. 4.9 – Gas in the collecting system. This is the film of an IVU sequence from a patient with a carcinoma of the bladder who, in addition to haematuria, complained of passing 'foam', with bubbles in his urine. A fistula had formed with the bowel, allowing gas to enter the bladder and the right ureter.

Having assimilated the notion of gas as the body's natural contrast agent for the purposes of diagnosis within the bowel, and evidence of the very serious situation of escape and leakage from it, it is now necessary to recognize and understand the significance of gas in the **wall** of certain structures, where it may occasionally be found (see below), e.g. the bladder.

Intramural gas may appear virtually anywhere of course, but in practice a commonly important place to look for it is the colon, e.g. in children.

Necrotizing enterocolitis

Look for (Fig. 4.10):

- Intramural colonic gas, especially on the right-hand side – note the dark margins forming a continuous track
- A normal appearing loop of bowel in the left flank with a normal wall of soft-tissue density contrasting with gas in the lumen
- Cardiac leads. Monitoring of the child reflects the severity of its condition. The child has also been intubated (note the endotracheal tube).

There are many causes of intramural gas, a list of which is given after several more examples (page 110).

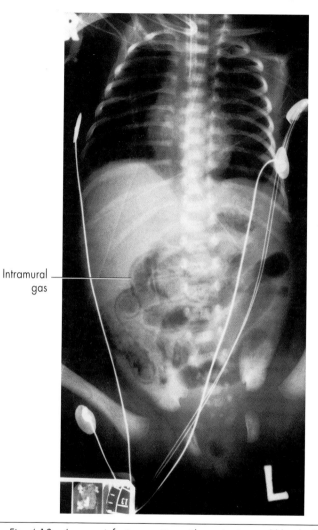

Intramural __ gas

L

Fig. 4.10 – A young infant presenting with prostration and bloody diarrhoea. Note the very clear edge of the colon outlined by gas in the wall of the bowel. This is necrotizing enterocolitis.

107

Pneumatosis coli

Look for (Fig. 4.11):

- Gas cysts protruding into the lumen of the large bowel causing a multiplicity of small pockets, far in excess of normal in the right upper quadrant
- Distortion of the normal mucosal pattern
- Evidence of perforation (not present here) – this may be localized or generalized, i.e. a pneumoperitoneum, or tracking into the mesentery. These 'poppings' of the gas cysts are usually benign but present with recurrent bouts of abdominal pain.

There may be an associated colitis in these patients and occasionally a psychiatric history.

Multiple gas cysts

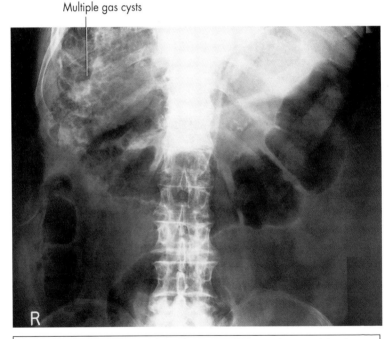

Fig. 4.11 – A 54-year-old woman with recurrent abdominal pain and diarrhoea. This is pneumatosis coli.

Gas in the bladder wall

Note (Fig. 4.12):

- The multiple irregular lucent pockets overlying the arc of the bladder outline
- This is 'emphysematous cystitis', associated with gas-forming organisms in the wall of the bladder
- A large rectal plug surrounded by gas can look similar, so careful analysis is necessary but the gas margin is usually smooth.

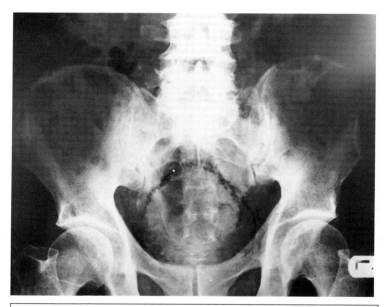

Fig. 4.12 – This is the lower abdominal X-ray of a 50-year-old man with severe urinary tract infection. The patient was diabetic.

Common

- Inflammatory bowel disease – may be a sign of impending perforation in toxic dilatation of the colon, a complication of ulcerative colitis
- Ischaemia of the bowel causing incipient necrosis/infarction, due to:
  - strangulation
  - volvulus
  - necrotizing enterocolitis
  - obstruction (premature infants)
- Pneumatosis cystoides. Usually benign. Often an incidental finding on X-ray (p. 108).

Rare

- Diabetes with infected gut wall (also gallbladder and urinary bladder)
- Iatrogenic (post endoscopy, biopsy, surgery)
- Obstructive pulmonary disease tracking down from chest (asthmatics, COPD patients)
- Peptic ulcer disease
- Penetrating injury
- Steroids (may be silent).

Approach to the problem

A **very high index of suspicion** must always be maintained for the possibility of intra-abdominal infection, especially in postoperative patients who do not recover quickly after surgery.

This is also true for patients who are just vaguely unwell but pyrexial on admission, as well as those with localizing signs.

Common major concerns are the subphrenic abscess after surgery, and pericolic abscess formation from rupture of the appendix or an infected colonic diverticulum, although these will usually be accompanied by pain. Penetrating injuries are also a potent source of transfer of bacteria into the abdomen (knives, bullets etc.), causing peritonitis.

Abscess formation leads to pus, and a large liquid collection may be readily detected by ultrasound or CT but remain only as a vague mass density or even undiagnosable on plain films. In the presence of gas-forming organisms, however, either multiple small bubbles or abnormal larger collections of gas and fluid may enable a plain film diagnosis of abscess formation to be suspected, and indeed the gas thus formed may block acoustic access and render the plain film superior to ultrasound for diagnosis in this regard, but not CT.

When an abscess is forming in a cavity the semisolid material mixed with gas bubbles may give it a granular texture like faeces, so caution must be exercised here. A good clue to the presence of an abscess is the **constancy of its position**, so 'look for the gas that has not moved' on serial films. Try to get erect or decubitus films with the affected side uppermost, in addition to supine films. Normal gut undergoing peristalsis causes changes in configuration minute by minute, although ileus may complicate the situation. Sentinel loops may appear around an abscess but will tend to lack mucosal folds. It is easy to mistake a fluid level in an abscess for just another loop of bowel in the early stages of its evolution.

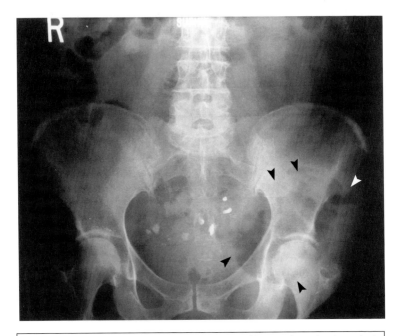

Fig. 4.13 – This is the supine AP film of a 72-year-old man admitted with marked left lower abdominal pain and tenderness. The patient was known to have extensive diverticular disease, most profuse in the sigmoid. This is an anterior abdominal wall abscess caused by tracking out to the left from an infected ruptured sigmoid diverticulum, which had eroded into the lower left overhanging (obesity) anterior abdominal wall.

Look for (Fig. 4.13):

- The large left-sided circular lucent area over the left hip, left iliac blade and left pelvic region. This is gas lying anteriorly in a large abscess cavity
- The multiple dense opacities in the pelvis – this is retained barium in diverticula from a previous enema, indicating that the patient has diverticular disease, and indicating a likely cause for the current problem
- The large gas–liquid level over the left hip region on the second erect film (Fig. 4.14). The weight of the fluid and general downward movement of structures in this position is typical. It is too big, high and lateral to be either a femoral or an inguinal hernia. Needle aspiration confirmed pus.

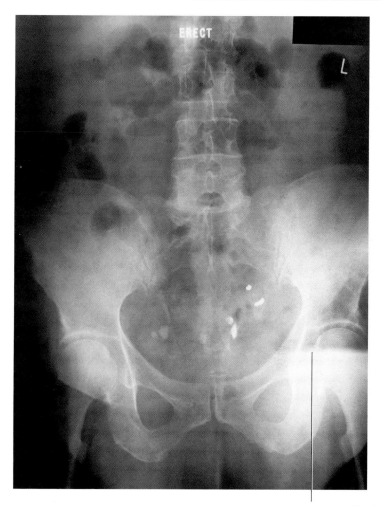

Gas-liquid level

Fig. 4.14 – Left lower anterior wall abscess (erect film).

NB Occasionally an abscess may form within a solid organ, creating a gas – liquid level, e.g. in the liver, spleen, and of course the brain.

Look at (Fig. 4.15):

- The gas collection under the right hemidiaphragm
- The associated fluid levels. This is pus in the abscess, indicating multiple loculi and an erect film
- The thinness of the right hemidiaphragm, indicating this is a 'naked diaphragm'
- The absence of any mucosal folds, supporting the conclusion that this is not part of the gut, i.e. colonic interposition, or interposed small bowel.
- Elevation of the right hemidiaphragm. This may or may not be present. 'Splinting' of the right hemidiaphragm may also occur, i.e. paralysis on screening, but 'screening of diaphragms' is now an antiquated concept and does not rule out a subphrenic abscess.
- Evidence of an associated pleural effusion or lobar collapse on the same side, which may or may not be present (not here).

Confirmation and imaging guidance for drainage may be carried out under ultrasound or CT control.

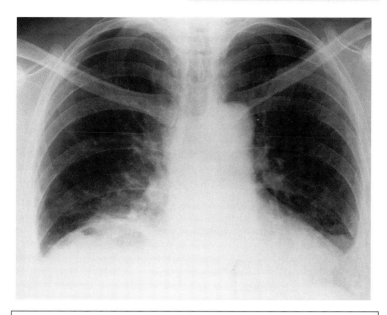

Fig. 4.15 – **Right subphrenic abscess** A 63- year-old woman who had a cholecystectomy carried out 8 days before, who is now pyrexial and tender in the right upper quadrant. This is a large right-sided subphrenic abscess.

Chapter 5

Ascites

The accumulation of free intraperitoneal fluid in the abdomen is an important clinical finding confirmed by the classic clinical sign of 'shifting dullness'. Radiologically a sign of massive free fluid includes distension of the abdomen.

In the supine position the bowel will tend to float on top of this pool of ascitic fluid and take up a central position. Some separation of the loops themselves may also occur because of the accumulation of fluid between them.

Also look for:

- A bulging shape to the abdomen
- A dense central grey part and sharp cut-off laterally, with dark flanks, due to the marked distension and abrupt change in curvature of the abdomen
- Greyness or 'ground-glass' appearance due to reduced contrast, and increased greyness caused by increased scattered radiation from the distension and fluid
- Medial displacement of the colon away from properitoneal fat stripes, of the inner abdominal wall. To be seen, this usually requires a bright light behind the film
- Loss of definition of liver tip, psoas margins, kidneys etc., due to surrounding fluid. As little as 7–10 ml of fluid may cause the liver tip to disappear
- Elevation of both hemidiaphragms (severe cases).

Causes of ascites

- Hypoproteinaemia (loss from gut or kidney)
- Cirrhosis of liver
- Congestive heart failure
- Inflammation (pancreatitis, tuberculous nodes)
- Malignancy with peritoneal metastases
- Lymphoma
- Occlusion of inferior vena cava

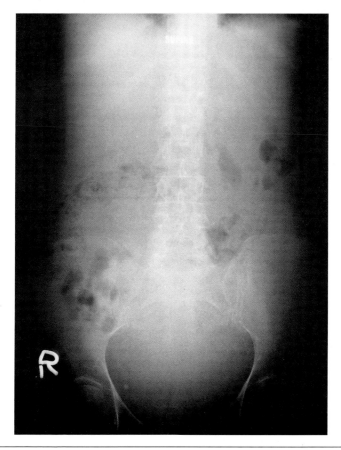

Fig. 5.1 – **Ascites** *Supine radiograph of a cirrhotic 48-year-old patient with centrally placed loops of small bowel and a distended abdomen. This is ascites.*

- Malnutrition
- Nephrotic syndrome
- Constrictive pericarditis.

Ascites usually starts to accumulate in the pelvis, tracks up the paracolic gutters, then gradually fills the abdomen.

Chapter 6

Abnormal intra-abdominal calcification

The causes of pathological calcification within the abdomen are many. Only the more common and important ones encountered in everyday clinical radiological practice will be described.

Abnormal vascular calcification

First remember that important medical conditions such as diabetes and chronic renal failure can cause premature vascular calcification – another good reason for checking the age of your patient both on the name badge from the date of birth and against any established degenerative changes in the spine.

Aorta/aortic aneurysms

If necessary, go back and revise the section on the normal aorta (pp 24–25). Get into the habit of looking for the aorta on *every* abdominal film, young or old. If necessary make it your 'favourite organ' (see hints at end of book).

Crucial fact: You must develop a very high index of suspicion for abdominal aortic aneurysm because this condition is so dangerous yet so potentially and eminently treatable by surgery or stenting, and it is frequently picked up as an incidental finding on plain abdominal X-rays.

The patient's life is then well and truly in the hands of those who see his films, and abdominal aortic aneurysms have repeatedly been missed on X-rays in the past, these patients subsequently dying suddenly when they ruptured.

If you learn nothing else from this book, learn to be ruthless in seeking out aortic aneuysms!! Ten seconds' searching may save the patient's life.

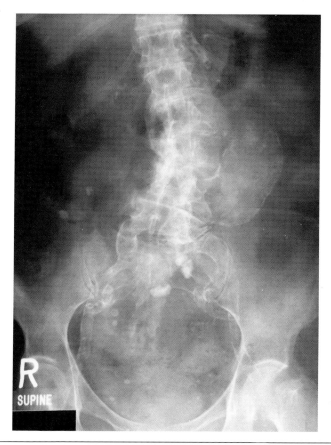

*Fig. 6.1 – **Aortic aneurysm** A 65-year-old diabetic and lifelong smoker. Note the large calcified mass bulging to the left. This is an abdominal aortic aneurysm.*

Look for (Fig. 6.1):

- The typical thin line of calcification in the wall of the aorta. Most aneurysms bulge to the left, but occasionally they may bulge to the right or symmetrically about the midline and still lie entirely over the spine
- Associated calcification in the iliac arteries, which is also present here. Aneurysms may form in these vessels as well.

Clinical/radiological problems

- The physician or surgeon may think he feels an aortic aneurysm in the abdomen and requests an X-ray 'to exclude it'. Thin patients, or patients with exceptionally lordotic spines, may well have a very palpable or 'thrusting' aorta, as may hypertensives, **so a normal aorta may simulate an aneurysm.**
- An obese patient may have a big aneurysm which cannot be confidently palpated, although you may be able to feel it when you know it is there!

NB Inability to palpate an aneurysm does not mean the patient has not got one. You should not be digging too hard anyway, in case you burst an undiagnosed aneurysm.

- Most aneurysms contain thin rims of calcification in their walls, but overlying gas, colonic material and X-ray scatter may make them very hard to find. The edge of the rim may lie just at the edge of the spine and be misinterpreted as part of the spine.
- Some aortic aneurysms have insufficient calcification in their walls to be seen, but normal anatomy may save the day.

Look for:

- A normally calcified aorta (patients over 40) over the spine with parallel or converging walls: this *does* exclude an aneurysm, but both walls must be unequivocally identified to do so.
Be aware, however, that not *every* body's aorta calcifies – even in the elderly.

Points to ponder: 1. Around 6 000 men die in the UK each year from ruptured abdominal aneurysms, and some of them have already had abdominal X-rays taken.
2. Albert Einstein died of a ruptured abdominal aortic aneurysm.

Other more complex problems

- The aorta may be tortuous or bent but not aneurysmal, an aneurysm in an artery being defined as loss of parallelism in its walls.
- Only one of the two walls of a tortuous but parallel-walled aorta may be visible – usually on the left, looking like an aneurysm when one is not present.
- A true aneurysm may have one wall bulging to the right of the spine – get used to looking for it here as well.
- Rarely some aneurysms are so large (e.g. > 8 cm) and their calcified walls so far apart and atypical that they go undetected if the observer is unaware of this phenomenon, or they may blend with the sacroiliac joints lower down.
- Most aneurysms are asymptomatic.
- Very rarely the superior mesenteric artery may calcify and, taking a long curved course to the left of the spine, may simulate an aortic aneurysm. In this situation, however, the aorta itself is likely to be calcified and should be visible as well.

Look at (Fig. 6.2):

- The thin rim of calcification to the left of L4 and distal to it
- The even more subtle rim of calcification to the right of L4 adjacent to the lumbar spine.

The patient had non-opaque gallstones. This was the typical incidental radiological presentation of an abdominal aortic aneurysm, or 'triple A'. It was missed by the first two doctors who looked at the film.

Look at (Fig. 6.3):

- The unequivocal focal expansion of the calcified wall of the abdominal aorta, confirming the presence of an aneurysm.

NB All images on X-rays are slightly magnified and this includes aneurysms, but aortas over 3 cm are usually regarded as aneurysmal. Some aortas can be >3 cm in diameter (so-called 'ectatic'), but *not* aneurysmal, so look for departures from parallelism, i.e. look at the shape of the aorta.

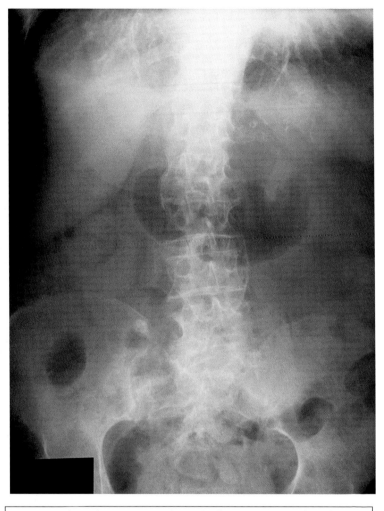

Fig. 6.2 – This is the supine AP radiograph of a patient X-rayed for right-sided abdominal pain. The first two doctors missed the aneurysm.

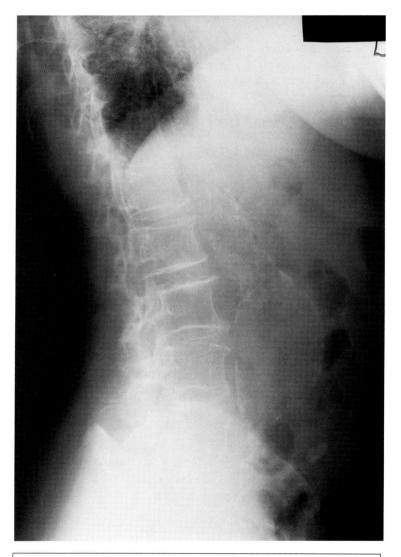

Fig. 6.3 – This is a lateral view of the same patient. The third doctor who saw the previous film was suspicious and requested this further view, confirming the diagnosis.

What To Do?

As in many other situations the answer to the radiological problem lies in requesting further views. Do not struggle on with just one film if you are not sure what is going on, but it is best practice to seek help before re-irradiating the patient unnecessarily. However, if you are alone and still unsure you may:

1. Request a lateral view of the abdomen. This will get the aorta off the spine and you will have a clearer mental picture of what you are looking at.
2. Request a supine left posterior oblique view (= right anterior oblique view). This is often superior to the lateral and gives an excellent view of the aorta in isolation from the spine, although you may find it harder to interpret. Radiologists, however, find this view extremely valuable. The solution to the possible presence of an aneurysm may therefore be solvable with plain X-rays, but ultrasound or abdominal CT are the next investigations of choice.

Is it leaking?

An early decision must be made with an acute abdomen as to whether to proceed straight to theatre or whether there is time to image the aorta, even with plain films.

Are the renal arteries involved?

If the aneurysm extends as high as L2 this is likely, but accessory renal arteries may be present at a lower level and can never be excluded by plain films. CT angiography, magnetic resonance angiography or conventional angiography may be necessary to confirm or exclude these.

Look at (Fig. 6.4):

- The irregular convex edges of calcification to the right of the lumbar spine
- The clear right psoas margin
- Loss of the left psoas margin and increased soft-tissue density on the left side with a convex edge further out to the left.

This is a leaking abdominal aortic aneurysm, with a haematoma accumulating in the retroperitoneum on the left side.

NB Clear psoas margins do not prove an aneurysm is not leaking if there is clinical evidence to the contrary.

NB Calcified lymph node

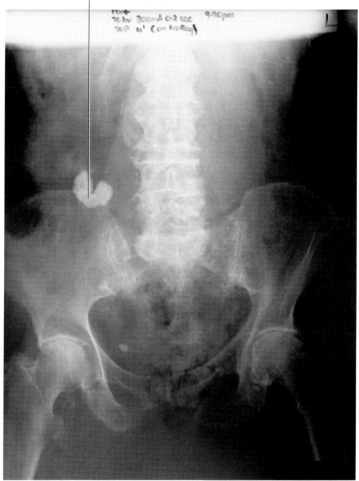

Fig. 6.4 – This is the abdominal X-ray of a 75-year-old woman admitted with severe abdominal pain and backache. The patient was in a state of shock with a rapid pulse and low blood pressure. This is a leaking aortic aneurysm. (NB the time at the top of the film. This is the sign of a very ill patient.)

? Leaking aortic aneurysm

Look for:

- A retroperitoneal mass effect with obliteration of the psoas muscle on one or either side
- Obliteration of one or other or both renal outlines
- Displacement of kidneys
- Displacement of the aorta by the haematoma
- Ileus in the gut
- Lumbar scoliosis
- The aortic aneurysm concave to the side of the leak which itself may or may not be visible.

Urgent ultrasound, or preferably spiral CT, should be carried out if there is time.

Non-urgent aneurysms should still be seen quickly by a vascular surgeon for further advice, depending on their size. The problem has then moved beyond the realm of plain films. Smaller aneurysms can be monitored every 6 months by ultrasound.

Other aneurysms: iliac/splenic/renal

Although a high index of suspicion must be maintained for abdominal aortic aneurysms in order to detect them, aneurysms in other vessels may also occasionally be seen.

Look for (Fig. 6.5):

- A biconvex calcified mass distal to the left or right of the point of division of the aorta at the inferior margin of L4
- Continuation of any aortic aneurysm distally, as here, into expanded iliac vessels. This is often (70%) the case, but not always so, and an iliac artery aneurysm can exist in isolation.

Remember: Although less common than abdominal aortic aneurysms, iliac artery aneurysms can kill you if they rupture. The diagnosis is readily confirmed with Doppler ultrasound if too much bowel gas does not intervene, or by CT/CT angiography. They are amenable to stenting or surgical repair.

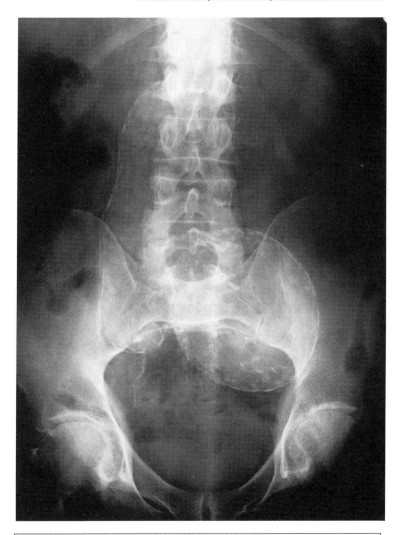

Fig. 6.5 – **Huge left iliac artery aneurysm** A 65-year-old man X-rayed for abdominal pain in whom an abdominal aortic aneurysm was found bulging to the right of the spine. Another calcified mass was noted in the left side of the pelvis. This is an iliac artery aneurysm.

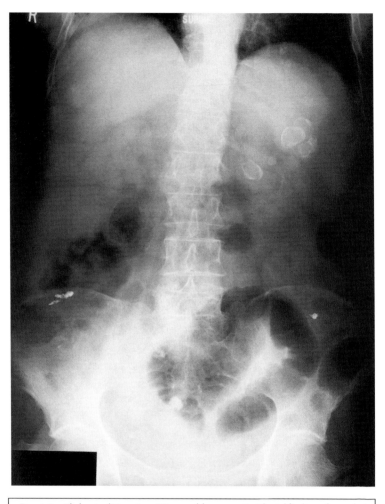

Fig. 6.6 – Abdominal X-ray in a 69-year-old woman. Incidental finding of rounded calcified masses in left upper quadrant. These are splenic artery aneurysms.

Splenic artery aneurysms

Look for (Fig. 6.6):

- The left/right marker. It is very easy when putting such films up to assume the patient has gallstones on the right, whereas these lesions are on the left. Check the L/R marker on every film you look at and *don't* put it up the wrong way round
- One or more circular or incompletely circular calcified masses in the left upper quadrant
- Splenic artery calcification. This may or may not be present.

Splenic artery aneurysms tend to be discovered incidentally on the X-rays of elderly patients, and are the second most common kind of aneurysm found in the abdomen, with about two-thirds containing calcification. They may also occur in young women and have a tendency to rupture during pregnancy, with a differential diagnosis of a 'ruptured ectopic' and a high mortality. They are usually asymptomatic and left alone in the elderly, but the opinion of a vascular surgeon may be sought. They may also occur in portal hypertension.

Renal artery aneurysms

These are rare and usually an incidental finding on imaging, but around one in five is bilateral. They may be associated with hypertension, pain and haematuria, and must be differentiated from renal calculi, gallstones etc. as they present as calcified rounded opacities in the flanks.

Causes of aneurysms

- Arteriosclerosis
- Hypertension
- Infection (mycotic)
- Trauma
- Congenital
- Fibromuscular dysplasia
- Polyarteritis nodosa.

NB The plain film detection of an aneurysm will usually lead to urgent further 'high-tech' investigations to confirm its presence and extent, but **the absence of a visible aneurysm on plain films does not mean the patient has not got one.**

Calcified lesions in the liver are relatively uncommon but occur from time to time. Of those that do, representative causes include:

- Old granulomas (TB, histoplasmosis)
- Primary liver tumours – hepatoma
- Secondary liver tumours, e.g. colloid carcinomas from the colon, ovary or stomach

  Hydatid cysts with fine lines or contracted edges if partially collapsed: the 'waterlily' sign.

Calcified gallbladder, chronic cholecystitis

Occasionally the gallbladder itself may calcify – 'porcelain gallbladder' – or the bile within it may be of high density – 'limey bile' – both these phenomena being associated with chronic cholecystitis.

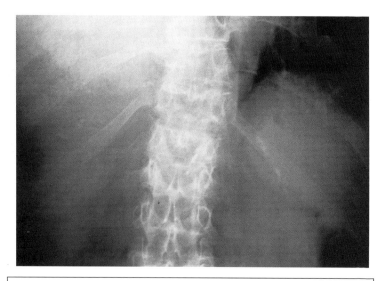

Fig. 6.7 – A 59-year-old patient with fine stippled calcification in the liver. This was secondary tumour from a colloid carcinoma of the colon. Note the associated elevation of the right hemidiaphragm due to liver enlargement.

Calcification in the spleen is an occasional and usually incidental finding on abdominal X-rays. It may vary from one or two specks of calcification to larger masses occupying almost all of the spleen itself.

Causes

- Cysts (congenital, post-traumatic, hydatid)
- Granuloma (old TB)
- Phleboliths (haemangioma)
- Infarction
- Parasites (*Armillifer armillatus*)
- Sickle cell anaemia.

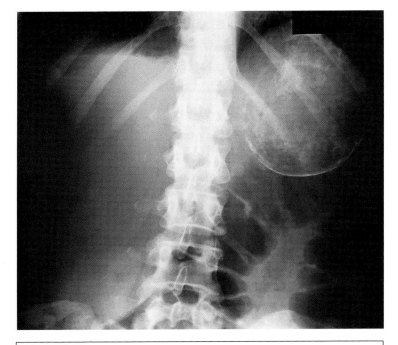

Fig. 6.8 – A 50-year-old woman. Incidental finding of calcified mass in spleen. This was a benign cyst but note the big liver.

Renal calculi (Fig. 6.9)

The majority of stones (85–90%) that form in the kidneys are radio-opaque, owing to their calcium content. They may range in appearance from multiple tiny opacities (nephrocalcinosis) to one big opaque stone completely filling the collecting system (staghorn calculus).

The plain film problem consists of proving that an opacity maintains a constant position in relation to one or other kidney by oblique films, erect films or control tomography, and differentiating between punctate costal cartilage calcification and gallstones, both of which are anteriorly placed structures, whereas kidney stones are posterior. Large stones may be confirmed to be posterior and therefore renal by a penetrated lateral view, even though they overlie the spine.

Other conditions, such as TB, cysts, tumours and renal artery aneurysms, may be associated with calcification, and non-opaque calculi can also occur, e.g. uric acid stones in gout. Renal stones may, sometimes, be demonstrated non-invasively by ultrasound and CT.

Some causes of renal calculi

- Hyperparathyroidism
- Infection
- Stasis/obstruction
- Dehydration
- Hypervitaminosis D
- Medullary sponge kidney
- Schistosomiasis
- Gout (uric acid stones).

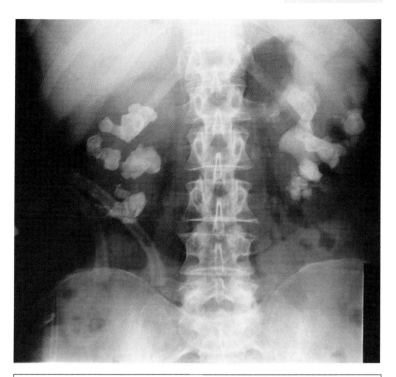

Fig. 6.9 – Abdominal X-ray. Staghorn calculus on left side. The right one is as yet incompletely formed. These can be treated by shock-wave lithotripsy and percutaneous extraction methods of interventional radiology.

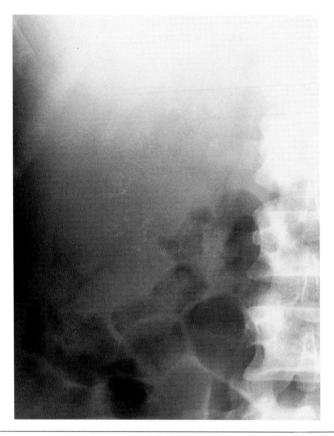

*Fig. 6.10 – **Nephrocalcinosis in right kidney** The left kidney had been removed.*

- In patients who present with suspected renal colic the hunt is on to find the obstructing calculus. Rarely other lesions, such as a sloughed papilla or blood-clot may cause obstructive symptoms, but first and foremost you are looking for a small calcified opacity in the line of the ureter.

- Cynics will tell you that all you can say about the ureter is that 'it goes from the kidney to the bladder', i.e. it may be tortuous, dilated and ectopic (and this is true), but the usual course is out of the kidney, up onto the psoas muscle, along the line of the tips of the transverse processes plus or minus a few millimetres, down over the pelvic brim and SI joints, round parallel to the lateral aspect of the true pelvis, then medially into the bladder above the level of the ischial spines.

Crucial fact: If you see such an opacity in a symptomatic patient do not assume it is an obstructing calculus, as many phenomena can mimic such a stone, e.g. costal cartilages, calcified lymph nodes, pelvic phleboliths etc. You must then request excretion urography (if the patient is not allergic to contrast medium) (a) for the radiologist to prove whether or not the opacity is an obstructing agent, (b) to confirm the level and constancy of the obstruction by serial films, and (c) to confirm whether or not the obstruction is complete.

The level will then dictate the management and approach to intervention, should this be required.

Remember: Emergency IVUs can take many hours to complete if the kidney is severely obstructed, because of delayed excretion. The examination is not complete until the level of the obstruction is established.

There are **three main positions** where ureteric stones are especially likely to obstruct:

- The pelviureteric junction
- The pelvic brim
- The ureterovesical junction.

What about allergic patients?

Renal ultrasound may show a dilated collecting system, and an ultrasound of the bladder may show a 'ureteric jet' of urine from the affected side, thus excluding obstruction of that ureter. Control CT scans of the abdomen may show oedema typical of an obstructed kidney and a calculus in the lower end of the ureter on the same side, thus avoiding contrast medium.

Megahint: If shown an IVU film in an exam always ask to see the control film: this is a film of the abdomen taken before any contrast medium is given. This will:

(a) Ensure that you do not miss an opaque calculus, which may 'disappear' completely after contrast is given (even a complete staghorn calculus), so you will not see it (see Figs 6.13 and 6.14);

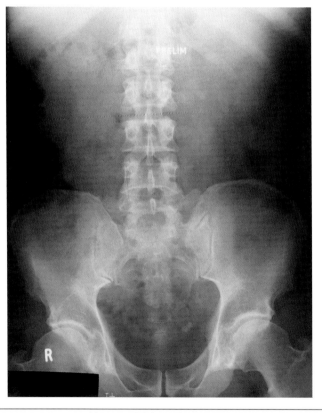

Fig. 6.11 – A 46-year-old man with left renal colic. Note the two opacities in the left side of the true pelvis. ? calculi.

(b) Impress the examiner and convey the fact that you understand IVU examinations and just exactly what you are trying to do.

Even if you are not shown a control film you will be given credit for asking for it.

NB A trainee radiologist in a radiology exam might be failed for not asking to see a control film, so this is a most important concept.

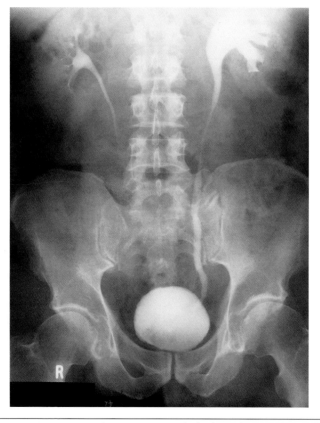

Fig. 6.12 – Same patient after contrast. Note the hydronephrosis and dilated left ureter down to the level of the opacities, confirming that these were obstructing calculi.

Value of control films.

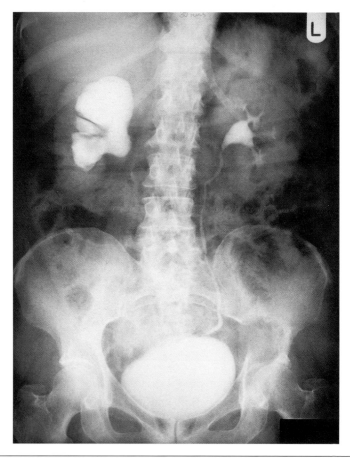

Fig. 6.13 – 30-minute post-contrast IVU film showing apparent large right staghorn calculus and normally excreting left kidney.

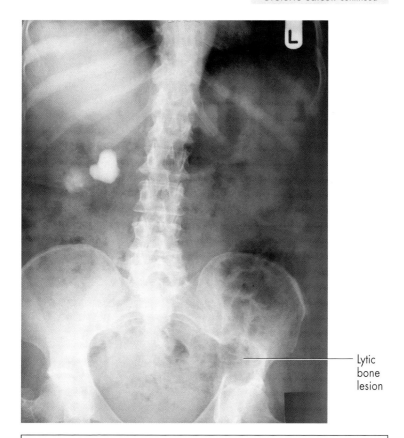

Lytic
bone
lesion

Fig. 6.14 – Control film on same patient before contrast, showing only a smaller obstructing calculus at the right pelviureteric junction and calcareous debris in the inferior calyx. Note also the lytic lesion in the left iliac bone. This patient had disseminated metastatic disease and hypercalcaemia, predisposing to renal stone formation.

Morals:

- The interpretation of a post-contrast film may be very different after its control film is seen.
- Be alert to the unexpected incidental finding and look right round the film for other abnormalities.

Stones in the bladder are relatively rare. They can be either large and solitary, e.g. the size of a hen's egg, or smaller, multiple and faceted. They may appear fortuitously in patients being X-rayed for other purposes, or be found in the bladder in patients being specifically investigated for urinary tract problems (dysuria, haematuria etc.).

Look for:

- A calcified object lying in the midline. In the supine position with a lot of urine in the bladder a heavily calcified stone will move to the dependent position, i.e. the posterior concavity of the bladder.
- Mobility. If you request right and left decubitus films mobility to the right and left dependent positions in a full bladder within its margins will confirm a bladder calculus (an ultrasound examination would, however, be preferable to avoid unnecessary radiation).
- Remember that a chronically inflamed bladder may be contracted round a stone and the patient unable to achieve bladder filling, precluding demonstration of this phenomenon.
- A bladder stone may actually be in a bladder diverticulum and therefore both eccentric from the midline and immobile on decubitus films. Further imaging tests would be necessary to confirm this (IVU, ultrasound, CT etc.).
- Occasionally a pelvic kidney can contain stones and fool you into misdiagnosing 'bladder stones'.

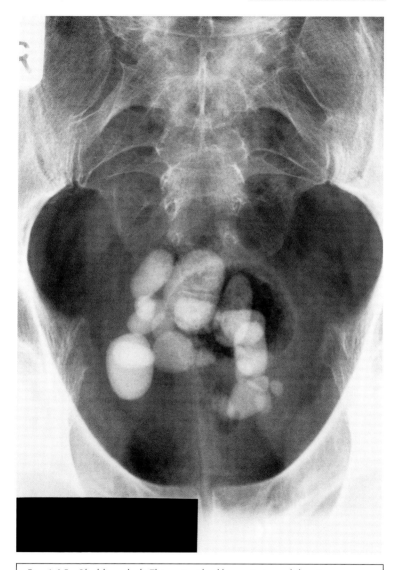

Fig. 6.15 – Bladder calculi. This patient had haematuria and dysuria.

Ureteric/bladder calcification

Something to be distinguished from luminal calculi in these structures is calcification in the walls of the ureters and/or bladder. This is a relatively rare phenomenon in UK patients with causes such as postradiation cystitis or neoplasms, but a very important and commoner radiological finding in certain other countries where schistosomiasis is endemic. Bladder calcification requires to be differentiated from calcified fibroids occupying its position and prostatic calcification in its base.

Causes

- Neoplasms
- Postradiation
- Tuberculosis
- Schistosomiasis
- Amyloidosis.

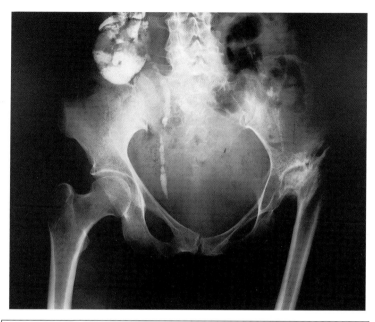

*Fig. 6.16 – **Calcified right ureter** A case of right-sided tuberculous autonephrectomy with calcification which has progressed down the right ureter. Note also the old left psoas abscess tracking down to the left hip joint, which has been entered and been partially destroyed by tuberculous disease from the spine. This also gave rise to a 'cold' abscess in the left groin. The disease on the right was arrested before it reached the bladder which did not calcify.*

Prostatic calcification ('calculi')

- In men aged 50 and over films of the abdomen and pelvis may begin to show punctate opacities appearing behind and above the symphysis pubis, caused by calcification in the prostate. This may be associated with infection, but this is not usually the case. It may be fine or coarse and occupy only part or all of the gland, so is not a reliable predictor of prostatic size.
- Prostatic calcification is not precancerous in itself, but it does not exclude malignancy in another part of the gland. The main differential is from a urethral calculus, which is usually midline in position, uniformly dense, smooth and solitary. Do not mistake the en-face soft-tissue shadow of the penis for a calcified bladder stone, prostate or urethral stone (see Misleading images and artefacts, page 176).

Hint: Do not mistake a melting suppository in the rectum for prostatic calcification!

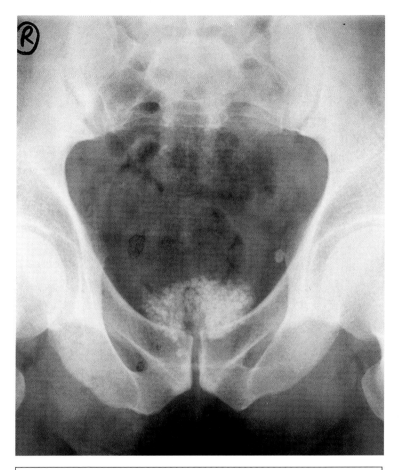

Fig. 6.17 – An example of calcification in the prostate. Note also the phlebolith adjacent to the left ischial spine.

Since only around 10% of biliary calculi are visible on X-rays, this is a poor way of looking for them. In patients who are clinically thought to harbour them, ultrasound is therefore by far the preferred initial method of investigation, and a negative film certainly does not exclude them. Nevertheless, patients will continue to present with opacities as an incidental finding in the right upper quadrant requiring clarification and occasionally a problematic ultrasound examination can be clarified with a plain film.

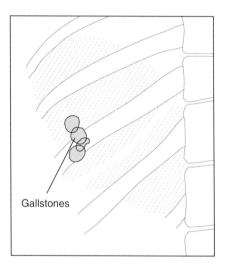

Gallstones

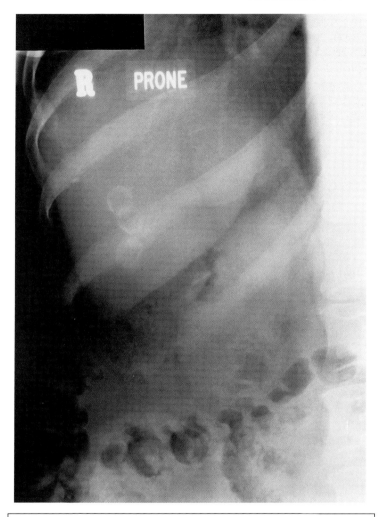

Fig. 6.18 – A cluster of opacities in the right upper quadrant in a middle-aged woman. These are gallstones.

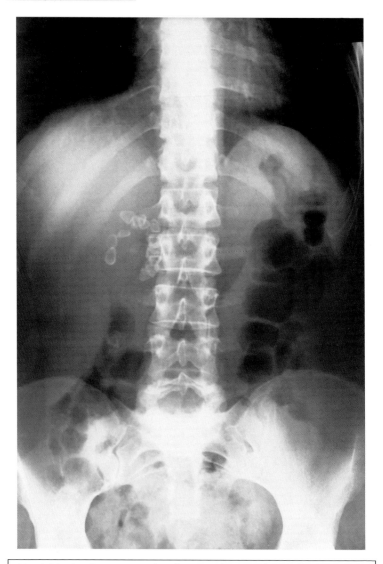

Fig. 6.19 – Another patient with gallstones in the cystic duct and bile duct. Note the Riedel's lobe extending over the right iliac crest (see p. 35).

Look for (Fig. 6.19):

- A single opacity or cluster of opacities in the RUQ or right flank. Gallstones may be single or multiple, large or very small. Their appearance may be very variable
- Evidence of a laminated or faceted structure, i.e. concentric rings or polygonal shapes due to abutment of stones one upon another
- Evidence of costal cartilage calcification/renal stone formation on both sides of the abdomen which may be mistaken for biliary calculi when seen on the right. But remember that renal and biliary stones can coexist, and the gallbladder lies in front of the right kidney.

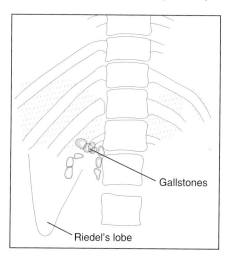

Gallstones

Riedel's lobe

Helpful hints

- Ask for a prone oblique right upper quadrant view. This will often isolate calculi in the gallbladder, especially if they are near the spine, and also cut down scatter from a full abdominal film, giving better clarity and contrast.

- Look lower down than just the right upper quadrant. The gallbladder may be low-lying because of a big liver, or be on a very long cystic duct. Occasionally it may even lie in the pelvis.

- A lateral view may help, as gallstones will tend to lie anteriorly and kidney stones posteriorly, but the film must be sufficiently penetrated.

- An erect abdominal film may cause small calculi to undergo 'layering', i.e. to form a small horizontal line as they float in the bile. The gallbladder may be contracted, however, and prevent this from happening if diseased or if the patient has just eaten.

- Remember that some stones are on the edge of visibility and by no means obvious and the vast majority (90%) are invisible anyway, due to a lack of calcified content.

These techniques may be helpful in demonstrating biliary calculi.

Pancreatic calcification

Look for (Fig. 6.20):

- Fine punctate foci of calcification lying from the right of the upper lumbar spine passing upwards and obliquely to the left to the region of the splenic hilum.

Remember:

- This may be very faint and difficult to see on plain films and may only show up on ultrasound, or particularly CT.

- The absence of visible pancreatic calcification does not exclude chronic pancreatitis.

- Calcification of the pancreas may also occur in cystic fibrosis, and occasionally with tumours.

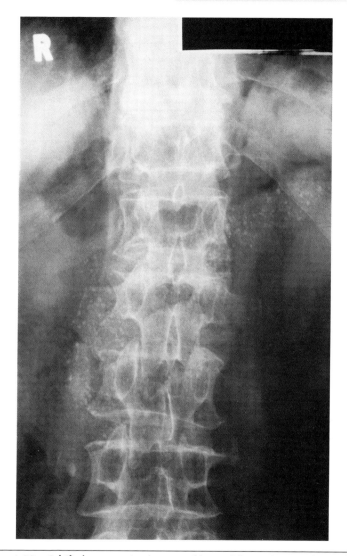

Fig. 6.20 – **Calcified pancreas** *Lumbar spine film. Middle-aged man with long history of alcoholism presenting with recurrent bouts of abdominal and back pain. This is a calcified pancreas, indicating chronic pancreatitis.*

See Figure 1.16. Incidental finding of extensive lymph node calcification, cause unknown. Note the potential difficulties if looking for coexistent renal or biliary calculi.

Because one or two calcified lymph nodes are so common on abdominal X-rays they are usually regarded as inert incidental findings without current clinical significance, but there are definite pathological causes.

Remember:

- Histoplasmosis
- Filariasis
- Lymphoma (post therapy) – especially retroperitoneal
- Calcifying metastases – thyroid, colon, osteosarcoma (rarely).

Megahint: Make sure you know whether or not the patient has had a lymphogram within the last year, as this will lead to persistently *opacified* but *not calcified* lymph nodes in the retroperitoneum, although they may look the same, owing to retained contrast medium. This, however, will progressively disappear over about 12 months but lymphograms are rarely done in the UK these days.

It is para-aortic and paracaval nodes that opacify at lymphography, i.e. only those over and adjacent to the spine. Those further out are usually in the mesentery, but mesenteric nodes can still lie over the spine.

The adrenals

The normal adrenals are not visible on plain abdominal X-rays, and tumours of these structures are only visible when significantly enlarged or calcified.

Patients with suspected adrenal disease should go directly to ultrasound, CT, MRI or radionuclide imaging. Calcified adrenals on plain X-rays mean little in terms of diagnosis, as most patients with calcified adrenals do not have Addison's disease, and vice versa. Nevertheless, it is instructional to recognize these for what they are and to understand the causes.

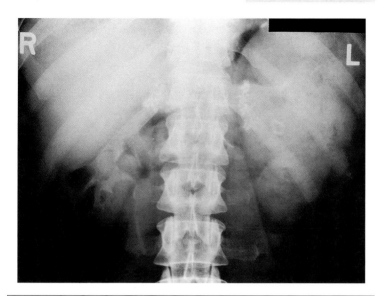

Fig. 6.21 –IVU film. There is faint excretion of contrast medium in the collecting systems. Incidental finding of bilateral adrenal calcification. The patient had no relevant symptoms or signs.

Bilateral adrenal calcification

Causes

- Haemorrhage (neonatal, perinatal or later), e.g. Waterhouse – Friederichsen syndrome
- Tuberculosis
- Histoplasmosis
- Amyloid
- Neoplasm, e.g. ganglioneuroma, carcinoma
- Phaeochromocytoma
- Wolman's disease (familial xanthomatosis)
- Addison's disease (rarely).

Chapter 7

The female abdomen

Apart from its distinct bony configuration being wider for the purposes of childbirth, certain pathological entities unique to the female pelvis may present themselves on plain abdominal X-rays. These consist primarily of masses with or without calcification, the configuration of the latter when present usually helping to narrow down the diagnosis.

NB The LMP of any woman of childbearing age should be known before subjecting her to irradiation of the abdomen. It should also be known to any observer who attempts to interpret any female patient's X-ray. Very rarely would a pregnant abdomen be deliberately X-rayed – e.g. after trauma or a 'one-shot' IVU. Tubal clips/or air-containing vaginal tampons may indicate that the patient has been sterilized or is undergoing the current LMP, respectively. The question 'Do you think you could be pregnant?', requires a firm negative before taking any X-rays.

Remember that one abdominal X-ray equals 28 chest X-rays or six and a half months of background radiation dose.

Causes of masses in the female pelvis

- Voluminous bladder (some women can hold up to 2 litres)
- Enlarged uterus (look for fetal parts/check LMP), consider haematocolpos in a young female child
- Uterine fibroid (calcified) (see Fig. 7.1)
- Ovarian masses. Benign cysts/neoplasms – may become very large and calcify
- Haematoma (after trauma)
- Abscess (postoperative) – look for pockets of gas
- Presacral meningocoele.

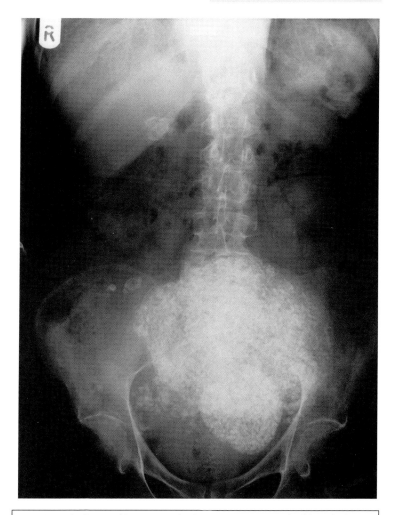

Fig. 7.1 – A 58-year-old woman with a huge craggy mass palpable in the lower abdomen. The X-ray shows heavy granular calcification. This is due to multiple adjacent uterine fibroids.
Note the incidental finding of gallstones in the right upper quadrant.

The preferred initial method of investigation of a pelvic mass in females is by ultrasound through a full urinary bladder. Transvaginal ultrasound may later be used as clinically indicated: this does not require a full bladder.

Wandering fallopian tube clips

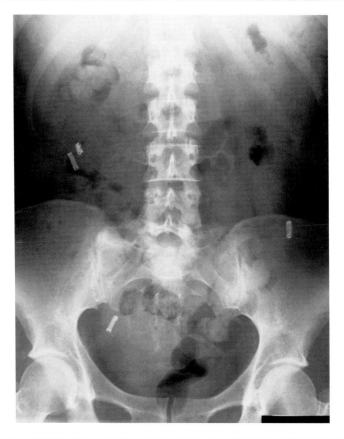

Fig. 7.2 – A woman of childbearing age in whom there had been several unsuccessful attempts at sterilization. If ultrasound cannot locate them, conventional radiography may still be required with due regard to the possibility of pregnancy.

Chapter 8

Abdominal trauma

Trauma to the abdomen may have important radiological manifestations which it is important to know about. These can be divided into penetrating injuries, such as knife or gunshot wounds to solid or hollow organs, or blunt impact trauma such as may occur in road traffic accidents. In these latter days of surgery and interventional radiology iatrogenic accidents may also occur within the abdomen, so that X-rays may be required to look for everything from malpositioned stents to retained swabs or forceps after operations.

Never think of abdominal trauma in isolation and to the exclusion of all else, but always as just one area of what may well be a multiply injured patient; conversely, if a head injury dominates the clinical picture, take full account of that but do not forget to consider that the abdomen and chest may have been injured as well, so examine both carefully and, if necessary, get them both imaged.

An early triage of the patient will of course be necessary to determine the best sequence of investigative procedures, but each trauma centre will have its own protocol.

In evaluating X-rays for abdominal trauma look for:

- The patient's **name**. Establish as quickly as possible the patient's identity for both medical and medico-legal reasons. Unconscious casualties may initially have to be labelled as 'unknown' or 'Mr X'. Get the name on the films as soon as possible, as multiple 'unknowns' may suddenly flood in, e.g. after a major motorway accident or rail crash, leading to potential mix-ups.
- The **time** of the film (e.g. 3.30 pm). Multiple serial X-rays may be required following admission and the subsequent temporal sequence may be important in following events, and the dates on all the films will be the same, unless they cross over midnight.

Also

- Check what is **left** and **right**. Do not mistake a normal liver for an injured spleen by failing to do this, or misdiagnose gas under the 'right; hemidiaphragm from seeing a normal stomach on a film you have put up back to front. (Note how frequently they do this on medical TV soaps, and even **real** medical programmes – occasionally even upside down!)

- Make good use of the **chest X-ray**, which will almost certainly have been taken as well; if not, then **request** one. This may help to resolve confusing upper abdominal findings, of both recent onset and pre-existing disease, as well as assisting the anaesthetist preoperatively.
- More than ever now is the time to look carefully at the **skeleton**, to check for **fractures** and **displacement** of bony structures. The confirmation of such findings will indicate the severity of injury and the likely organs involved, e.g. left lower ribs: spleen; and pelvic bones: the bladder.

Look for:

- Free gas in the peritoneal cavity. This will indicate the rupture of a hollow viscus or a penetrating injury of part of the gut, indicating the necessity for urgent surgery. Do not forget that colonic interposition and other phenomena may mimic a pneumoperitoneum, but look for the 'double-wall sign' (see page 89) as well as for air under the diaphragm. Remember: seriously ill patients may not be fit for erect films, in which case a left or right decubitus view may be attempted and free gas sought in the flanks, but all the diagnostic work-up may have to be done on **supine** films alone if the patient is not fit even for this, so familiarize yourself with the **supine manifestations of free air** for this eventuality (see section on pneumoperitoneum, p. 89).
- Gas in the retroperitoneum. (See Chapter 4, p. 100). A stab in the back or retroperitoneal rupture of the bowel may occur without visible air in the peritoneal cavity. Look for irregular outlines of dark air densities around the psoas muscles, kidneys and diaphragmatic margins.
- Apparent enlargement of normal organs such as the liver, spleen and kidneys – this may indicate subcapsular haematoma formation or even rupture of these organs, especially if their normal outlines have been lost. Such collections can be massive and can be diagnosed by displacement of the bowel from lack of normal gas in these locations.
- Loss of the psoas margins. When this is seen in the context of trauma it is likely to represent a massive retroperitoneal haematoma, indicating severe injury and blood loss. Look for fractures in the transverse processes, scoliosis concave to the injured side, and evidence of bony injuries in the lowermost ribs.

- Be aware that trauma can cause secondary ileus and a large accumulation of gas, which can interfere with trauma assessment.
- Displacement of hollow organs, e.g. the stomach medially and downwards with an enlarging spleen, or upward displacement of small bowel loops out of the pelvis with a ruptured bladder. Check also for an overloaded bladder and catheterize the patient, if not already done, to relieve this and monitor possible haematuria and urine output subsequently.
- Foreign bodies, e.g. bullets in the USA and other countries where guns are freely available.

Crucial facts to remember

- A normal initial X-ray does not exclude significant intra-abdominal trauma.
- X-rays are just one modality in the imaging armamentarium used in trauma, although in some parts of the world they may be the only one.
- Urgent and early ultrasound – or better, CT scanning – may be preferable to save time in critically injured patients in evaluating, for example, the liver and spleen, and remember that delayed rupture of the spleen in particular can occur. Injury to the pancreas leading to traumatic pancreatitis may often be uncovered by CT, and colour Doppler ultrasound may confirm or exclude perfusion of organs and limbs.
- The head, chest, abdomen and limbs can be rapidly scanned in a spiral CT machine, although essential immobilization/anaesthetic devices may slow things down a bit.
- Early progress to excretion urography, urethrography or arteriography may be an urgent and necessary follow-on from plain X-rays in the evaluation of trauma.
- MRI may be urgently required to assess spinal trauma.
- **Do not unnecessarily take out a patient's functioning kidney: he may only have the one.** You must make every effort to establish the presence or otherwise of another working kidney before taking out the only one he or she has, and remember that kidneys have remarkable powers of regeneration. And consider this for any injured kidney: 'Would I still take out this injured kidney if I knew it was the only one?'
- **Do not waste time with imaging if the patient is bleeding to death in front of you.** Resuscitation must come first, and after that in some cases immediate

transfer to theatre may be required, and if necessary X-rays undertaken only then at the discretion of a senior doctor.

Trauma: ruptured kidney

Note (Fig. 8.1):

- The swelling of the right kidney
- The escape of contrast from the right collecting system, indicating rupture of the kidney. A large volume of blood is escaping as well.
- The scoliosis concave to the injured side (indirect sign)
- And most importantly: another normally excreting kidney on the opposite side.

Footnote: Escape of contrast like this can occur in severe renal obstruction in the acute setting, or also in the chronic setting where it can form a huge retroperitoneal fluid collection called a 'urinoma'.

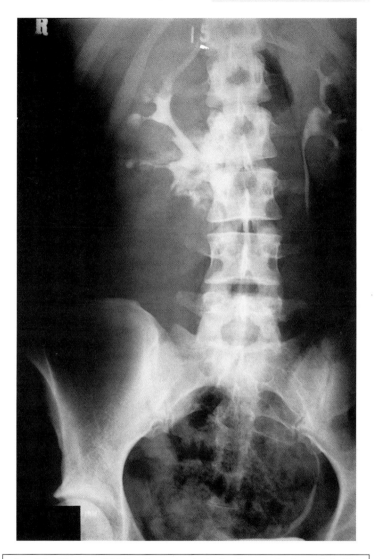

Fig. 8.1 – This is an IVU film of a patient kicked in the right flank in a fight. The plain film showed loss of the right renal and psoas outlines.

Old trauma

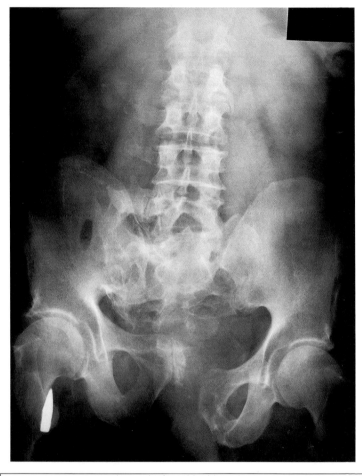

Fig. 8.2 – AP supine radiograph of an old soldier who 'stopped one' during the Normandy campaign in 1944. The left pubic ring and right sacral wing had been smashed by the bullet, which then tumbled and came to rest beside the right femur in the groin. Evidence of old trauma may occasionally present on abdominal films causing confusing bone changes.

Look for (Fig. 8.3):

- Complete separation of the lower thoracic spine and corresponding ribs
- Rupture of the left hemidiaphragm with separation from the chest wall
- Fractures of the upper ribs and bilateral surgical emphysema
- Colon in the chest
- Left basal pneumothorax
- Displacement of the heart to the right
- Sandbags stabilizing the head.

The child died from coexistent severe head injuries.

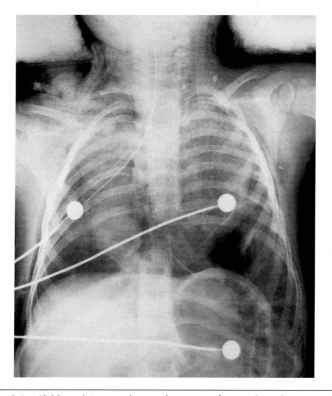

Fig. 8.3 – Child aged 4 years who was thrown out of a car when it hit a tree. No seat belt. Suffered severe multiple injuries and killed.

Chapter 9

Iatrogenic objects

Radiological

In this age of well-developed interventional procedures in radiology it is common to see objects that have been deliberately placed in the abdomen to treat disorders in most systems. Being able to recognize some of these for what they are will enable you to deduce what has been wrong with and done to your patients. The position of these devices may also be monitored by plain X-rays to confirm that they are still in position and have not slipped, leading to malfunction.

Typical devices to look for include:

- Aortic/iliac stents for vascular stenoses – with wire mesh structures in the line of arteries
- Biliary/urinary/GI tract stents for stenoses – oesophagus/rectum/sigmoid
- Temporary nephrostomy tubes to decompress obstructed kidneys often with pigtails to aid position retention
- Abscess drainage tubes
- Inferior vena cava filters (to prevent pulmonary emboli from the legs)
- Embolization coils/balloons – to ablate vessels in tumours prior to or as an alternative to surgery, and to shut down pathological circulations.

Retained contrast medium

This may also be seen in the appendix or colonic diverticula (barium) and in the spinal canal (myodil) — with round blobs of this high density agent from previous myelography examinations. It may even extend right up to the head.

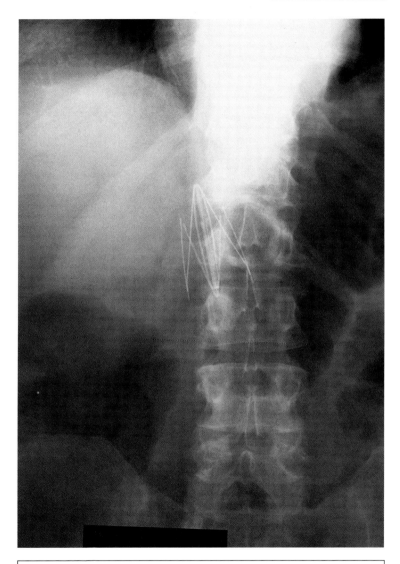

Fig. 9.1 – Inferior vena cava filter.

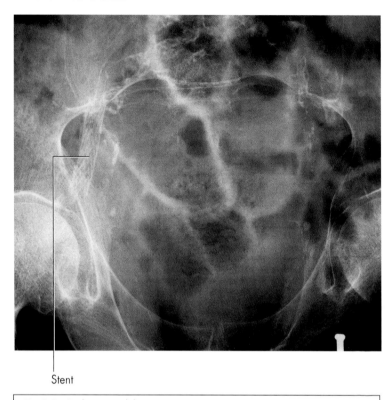

Stent

Fig 9.2 – Right external iliac stent.

A host of other objects associated with past or current therapy or previous surgery may also present themselves on abdominal X-rays.

Look for:

- Surgical sutures or clips, often tiny and hard to see unless made of dense material
- Nasogastric tubes in the stomach (usually with an opaque tip). These can curl up in the nose, pharynx or oesophagus, back-track up the oesophagus, or get knotted in the stomach! They may even be lying down the right or left main bronchus! Get views of the head or neck if the tubes have not reached the stomach
- Small opacities over buttock areas (previous bismuth injections or crystalline penicillin for VD etc.)
- ECG leads – upper abdomen/lower chest
- Wires from TENS machines to control pain
- Cutaneous patches (nicotine, hormones etc.)
- Ventriculoperitoneal shunts (hydrocephalus) – don't mistake for nasogastric tubes! They often lie over the medial lung fields and are outwith the stomach.
- Syringe driver tubes (morphine etc.)
- Pacemakers
- Tantalum gauze (previous surgical repairs – groin/umbilicus)
- Pessary rings – uterine prolapse.
- Fallopian tube clips
- Radioactive seeds, e.g. in pelvis
- Metal hip prostheses from previous fractures to the neck of the femur
- Prosthetic heart valves – sometimes visible on upper part of abdominal films
- Umbilical catheters (children)
- Bladder catheters
- Intrauterine contraceptive devices (pelvis)
- Recently ingested pills.

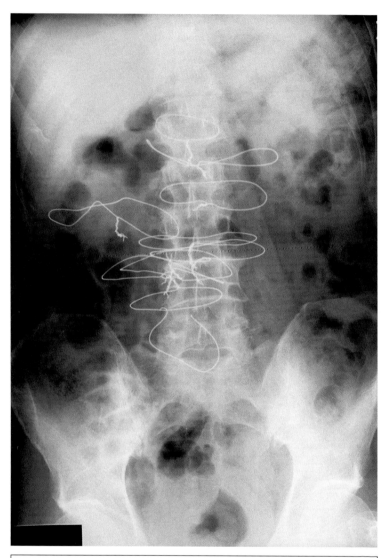

Fig. 9.3 – This patient had very strong steel sutures put in for an anterior abdominal wall incisional hernia.

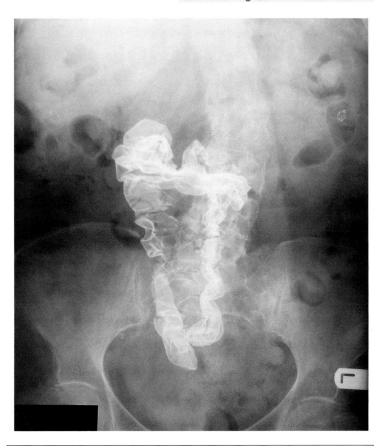

Fig. 9.4 – More 'surgical footsteps'! Tantalum gauze used to treat a ventral hernia. Sometimes it can also be found in the groin for herniorrhaphy repairs. It breaks up with time. Don't mistake it for a retained swab!

Chapter 10

Foreign bodies, artefacts, misleading images

There is no end to the list of foreign bodies that may end up inside a patient's abdomen, and this is particularly true of children. Typically ingested objects include coins, beads, ball bearings, toys, safety pins, ring-pulls, mercury batteries etc. Some foreign bodies will be poorly seen, e.g an aluminium ring-pull, and some may be completely invisible, such as a small rubber ball.

It is important to view the child as a whole and not simply the stomach in isolation, that is, the ears, nose, mouth and pharynx should be checked clinically, and any history of stuffing foreign bodies into any other orifices, as well as swallowing them, should be sought, or even other children's orifices!!

Depending on the timescale it may be expedient to X-ray the child from the level of the nasopharynx to the rectum in one go, as a foreign body may lodge temporarily in the lower oesophagus and may be missed if only an abdominal X-ray is taken.

Later, when the child feels discomfort in the lower oesophagus but the foreign body moves into the stomach, it may be missed on a chest X-ray taken later – only to pass on when it has apparently been 'excluded' but between the temporal sequence of the two films has actually been missed. Due regard to minimizing radiation dose must, however, be constantly borne in mind. But X-rays may be necessary to prove a foreign body has passed.

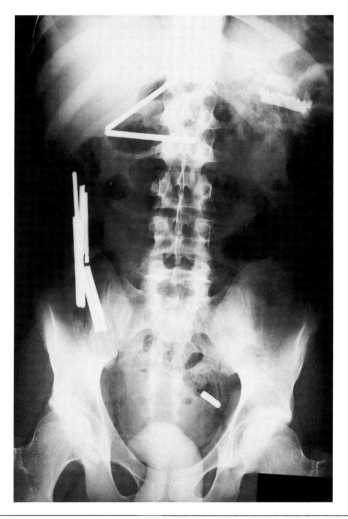

Fig. 10.1 – Psychiatric patient who enjoyed meals of mercury and glass thermometers. Note also the razor blade in the left upper quadrant – these are usually wrapped in sellotape by the patient, but are not visible radiologically. The nurses in this patient's ward got into trouble because thermometers kept disappearing. The chest X-ray showed multiple small mercury globules which had been inhaled into the lungs when the patient crunched the thermometers.

Adults, especially if subnormal, may ingest all manner of strange objects, and of course insert all manner of objects into their rectums.

Criminals and drug smugglers may swallow sachets of heroin or other drugs, or stuff them in their children's soft toys.

Occasionally multiple small speckled opacities may be seen in the abdomen. These can be anything from pica (dirt, stones etc.), eggshells, broken dental fillings, to lead paint – the latter having diagnostic significance when lead poisoning is being sought.

Apart from entertainment value the most important fact to consider with an ingested foreign body is, will it pass spontaneously (e.g. a small ball bearing) or will it not (e.g. an open safety pin)? The decision must then be made whether to wait, watch and review (if necessary with a follow-up X-ray), or intervene endoscopically or surgically to retrieve it. Psychiatric advice may also be appropriate in some cases.

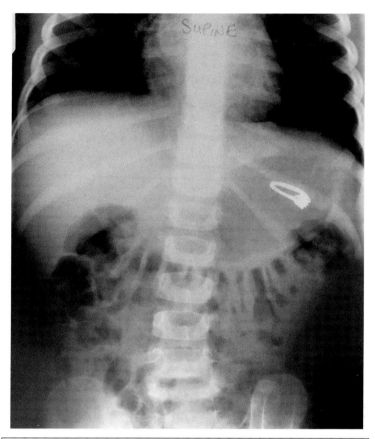

Fig. 10.2 – Engagement ring swallowed by young child. The insurance company would not pay up as the owner 'knew where it was' and so by definition it was not lost. Should pass spontaneously. The diamonds, being real, did not show up as they are made of carbon!

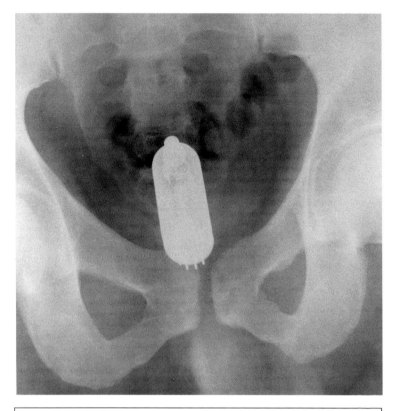

Fig. 10.3 – An adult male presenting with rectal pain and bleeding. This object was an old-style glass radio valve which he claimed to have 'sat on', as such patients often do. It was impacted distally into the anal mucosa by its prongs.

The main problems are:

- How to extract the foreign body without breaking it or lacerating the mucosa
- Minimizing the danger to yourself regarding HIV, hepatitis, septicaemia etc.
- Minimizing the danger to the patient
- Controlling your own and your staff's mirth in dealing with such a patient – you must learn to keep a straight face in such circumstances, and be sympathetic towards the patient's embarassment and plight.

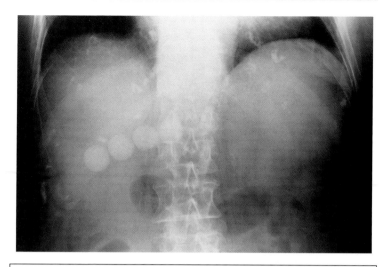

Fig. 10.4 – Elderly patient presenting with right upper quadrant pain and suspected calculous cholecystitis. Note the four opacities in line in the RUQ.

Note:

- These are all identical in size, shape and density.
- Gallstones are never so perfect. ?Artefacts.

These turned out to be pandrops in a bag in the patient's pocket! The opacities had gone after the bag of sweets was removed for the repeat film. Note the punctate costal cartilage calcifications.

NB The patient could still have had cholecystitis with non-opaque gallstones and still required investigation.

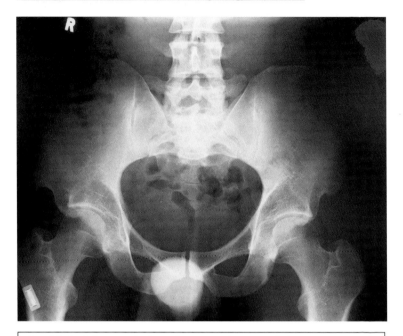

Fig. 10.5 – Soft tissue shadow of penis simulating a calculus in a young male patient. Learn to recognize this to avoid making a fool of yourself by asking what it is on the ward round. Another example is shown in Fig. 1.2.

Chapter 11

The acute abdomen

Causes

The most important causes of an acute abdomen which may be associated with plain film radiological signs include:

- Perforated viscus (especially a duodenal ulcer, but any part of the GI tract may rupture), with peritonitis
- Ruptured aortic aneurysm
- Renal colic
- Biliary colic
- Acute cholecystitis
- Acute pancreatitis
- Acute appendicitis
- Intestinal obstruction
- Acute diverticulitis
- Volvulus
- Hernias
- Abscesses
- Vascular occlusions
- Intussusception
- Toxic dilatation of colon.

Do not forget, however, to view the patient as a whole to take a **chest X-ray** and remember that

- Myocardial infarction
- Basal pneumonia
- Dissecting aorta
- Pulmonary embolism etc. may all masquerade as an acute abdomen.

Remember also that the radiological signs may not be present or fully evolved at the time of presentation, so if necessary re X-ray the patient after an hour or so, or move on rapidly to ultrasound, CT, IVU, angiography or whatever is appropriate to establish the diagnosis without delay.

Oral water-soluble contrast or rectal contrast may be given to confirm or exclude visible evidence of leakage or obstruction in appropriate circumstances, but this should only be after discussion with the radiologist.

Remember also the many causes of acute lower abdominal pain due to gynaecological disorders in women, e.g. dysmenorrhoea, salpingitis, ovarian cyst torsion etc.

Remember in addition to the above common medical conditions that simulate an acute abdomen the other rarer medical causes of acute abdominal pain, such as porphyria, Addisonian crisis, diabetic crisis, and lead poisoning etc.!

Chapter 12

Hints

- Never forget to check the name and the date first and get all the other data you can off the name badge. Films can easily get in the wrong packets!
- Check male or female.
- Check left and right.
- Make sure everything is on the film, from the hemidiaphragms to the inguinal canals, or covered by several films.
- Make sure you understand how the film was taken, i.e. erect, supine, decubitus, or oblique, and that you understand the implications of each position and what to expect, e.g. fluid levels do not appear on supine films.
- You see what you look for — don't underestimate the 'mark 1 eyeball'!
- In acute abdomens always get a chest X-ray, preferably erect. Remember that serious chest disease may mimic serious abdominal disease, and vice versa, secondary X-ray changes to abdominal disease may occur in the chest.
- Check the lung bases and look for the breasts on abdominal films.
- Find the faeces and you've found the colon.
- Acquire previous films as soon as possible to compare with new ones.
- Make sure you've put the film up the right way round!
- Only view films under proper conditions of illumination, i.e. on a viewing box, waving them in front of a window on a ward round will guarantee you will miss 20% of what there is to see.
- Put a bright light behind any area too dark to see properly on the viewing box. Sod's Law will always conceal a significant abnormality in a very dark area e.g. rib fractures.
- You must be able to explain everything you see on a film in terms of anatomy, pathology, or artefacts.
- Do not ignore something you do not understand: work out what it is or go and ask someone else who can help you – and in a seriously ill patient, do it **early**.
- Do not be too proud or self-conscious to seek help early.
- 'Nothing excludes anything' is a good working aphorism. Life-threatening

illness may be present with no or only a few radiological signs.

- 'Rules are for the obedience of fools and the guidance of wise men', i.e. do not stick slavishly to protocols. Adjust your actions appropriately to the patient's problems, and keep a global view of the patient at all times.
- When in doubt, do the right thing. Like calling a radiologist at 2 a.m.
- 'Every woman is pregnant until proved otherwise'. Get the LMP before requesting X-rays.
- Keep an open mind. Remember the concept of differential diagnosis.
- Do not be boxed in by other peoples' suspected labels and diagnoses.
- Learn to work out the age of patients from the appearance of their films (i.e. from vascular calcification, degenerative spinal changes, cortical thinning, times of epiphyseal closure etc.), and cross-check it with the date of birth and the date the film was taken.
- Maintain a sceptical outlook on all data supplied. Left/right markers can be incorrect and the wrong names get on patients' films. 'Check for gross error.' Your patient may deny previous surgery but have wire sutures visible. Have you got somebody else's film in your hand, or is your patient demented?
- Learn to look, think and articulate/discuss the findings on X-ray films simultaneously. This takes many years to perfect, but now is the time to start.
- Minimise the radiation dose to patients by taking no more films than necessary.
- To see *fluid levels* you need *fluid*, *gas* and an *erect* or *decubitus* film, with a horizontal X-ray beam. Supine films are done with a vertical beam.
- Do not create chaos by misinterpreting tantalum gauze as a retained swab.
- Beware of bowel gas. It can hide any abnormality and simulate lytic bone disease.
- Always remember that your clinical diagnosis may be *wrong*. Do not develop an ideé fixé every time you look at a film. Remember the concept of *differential* diagnosis and be receptive to information which may contradict your first impression on the X-rays.
- The patients don't read the textbooks — they will not always present with all the symptoms and signs of a particular condition.
- Practise looking at X-ray films in books, journals, computer programmes, the Internet etc. and 'present' them verbally to yourself or other medical students/colleagues until this becomes second nature.
- Do not have a passive attitude to radiographs. If they are technically unacceptable get them repeated, as long as it is clinically justified .
- Understand the limitations of X-ray films: serious disease can still be present

with a negative film, but someone else may see signs which you have not seen. By definition we do not know what we have missed – until the post mortem! The same film can look dramatically different on another occasion, or if just a little bit more clinical information is supplied or another view is taken.

- Remember that X-rays do not provide answers in every case.
- Learn to identify a calcified aorta over the spine, whether normal or aneurysmal. This must become a reflex.
- In everyone over 40 check for Aneurysms, Aneurysms, Aneurysms – the 'triple A' of ER, i.e. 'Abdominal Aortic Aneurysms'. You may save the patient's life.
- Pick a favourite organ in the abdomen that you look for especially in every patient.
- Look critically at iatrogenic objects such as nasogastric tubes. Do not assume that because they were put in by 'experts' they are in the right place. Often they are not, or they may have moved. Check against previous films.
- Small fluid levels can occur normally.
- Get a history of any previous surgery before trying to interpret any X-ray film and make sure you record it on the request for the radiologist.
- Do not mistake a stoma for an abnormal mass.
- If time allows, re X-ray the patient after a period of time, to allow any radiological changes to evolve. Do not waste time with abdominal X-rays in critically ill patients. If indicated, go straight to abdominal CT scanning or theatre for immediate surgical intervention (e.g. ruptured aortic aneurysm).
- Do not sit back and wait for something to jump out at you from the film and if nothing does so call it 'normal'.
- Learn the radiological signs of abnormality then go looking for them.
- Milk the film you've got before asking for another one.
- The diagnosis of normality is an important conclusion to arrive at and is the one the patient most wants to hear.
- Go and see the radiologist early with difficult films.
- Be alert to incidental findings, especially outwith your main area of interest. These may be of even greater importance to the patient than that which you are looking for. Remember that aortic aneurysms are usually found incidentally.
- Beware of steroids. These drugs increase the likelihood of GI tract perforation and also mask the signs.
- Write X-ray request forms clearly, legibly and provide accurate, full and all

relevant clinical information. This will enable the radiologist to optimize the diagnostic value of the films you have requested. Print your name and give your bleep and ward number clearly, so the radiologist can contact you back with urgent findings. Patients have died because doctors' names were illegible on X-ray forms. Inadequate and illegible requests are dangerous, misleading, annoying and negligent.

- Memorize a template so that you can present any X-ray case verbally. For example: 'This is an *abdominal X-ray* of *Margaret Smith* taken on *9 September 2001* when she was *75 years old*. The positive finding is *distended small bowel* and this is consistent with a differential diagnosis of *obstruction* and *ileus*, of which the most likely is *obstruction*.' Fill in the underlined parts depending on your findings.

Then wait for the cross-examination.

And finally:

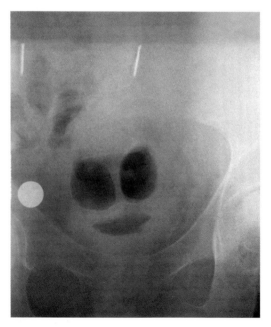

Stay cool!

Index